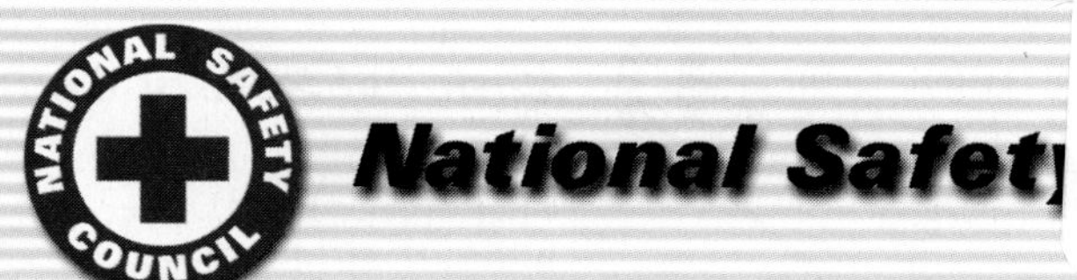

CPR

Fourth Edition

Alton Thygerson, Ed.D.
Consultant/Medical Writer
National Safety Council

JONES AND BARTLETT PUBLISHERS
Sudbury, Massachusetts
BOSTON TORONTO LONDON SINGAPORE

JONES AND BARTLETT PUBLISHERS

40 Tall Pine Drive, Sudbury, MA 01776
978-443-5000
nsc@jbpub.com
http://nsc.jbpub.com

Jones and Bartlett Publishers Canada
2406 Nikanna Road
Mississauga, ON L5C 2W6
CANADA

Jones and Bartlett Publishers International
Barb House, Barb Mews
London W6 7PA
UK

National Safety Council®
Emergency Care Programs
1121 Spring Lake Drive
Itasca, IL 60143-3201
(630) 285-1121
(800) 621-6244
www.nsc.org

Executive Director, Home & Community Safety and Health Group: Donna Siegfried

Program Development & Training Manager, Home & Community Safety and Health Group:
Barbara Caracci

Production Credits
Chief Executive Officer: Clayton E. Jones
Chief Operating Officer: Donald W. Jones, Jr.
Executive V.P. and Publisher: Tom Manning
V.P. and Managing Editor: Judith H. Hauck
V.P., Sales and Marketing: Paul Shepardson
V.P., Production and Design: Anne Spencer
V.P., Manufacturing and Inventory Control: Therese Bräuer
Publisher, EMS & Aquatics: Lawrence D. Newell
Emergency Care Senior Acquisitions Editor: Tracy Foss
Director of Marketing, EMS and Health Sciences: Kimberly Brophy
Emergency Care Associate Editor: Jennifer Reed
Production Editor: Linda S. DeBruyn
Interactive Technology Director: W. Scott Smith
Text Design: Studio Montage
Typesetting and Editorial: Nesbitt Graphics
Illustrations: Rolin Graphics
Interior Photos: Richard Nye
Cover Design: Studio Montage
Cover Photographs (clockwise from top left):
© Brian Pieters, Masterfile;
© Wedgworth, Custom Medical Stock Photo;
Photo courtesy of Heatstream;
Richard Nye
Additional Photographs:
Chapter 1 - © Mark E. Gibson
Chapter 2 - © Jeff Albertson/Stock, Boston/PictureQuest; Figure 1 Courtesy of The American Academy of Orthopaedic Surgeons
Chapter 3 - © 1998 Bob Winsett, Index Stock Imagery, PictureQuest; Figure 6 Courtesy of The American Heart Association
Chapter 4 - © Custom Medical Stock Photo
Chapter 5 - © IT STOCK INT'L, Index Stock Imagery, PictureQuest
Printing and Binding: Courier Company

The CPR procedures in this book are based on the most current recommendations of responsible medical sources. The National Safety Council and the publisher, however, make no guarantee as to, and assume no responsibility for, the correctness, sufficiency or completeness of such information or recommendations. Other or additional safety measures may be required under particular circumstances.

Printed in the United States of America
05 04 03 02 10 9 8 7 6 5

About the National Safety Council Program

Congratulations on selecting the National Safety Council's First Aid and CPR program! You join good company, as the National Safety Council has successfully trained over 6 million people worldwide in first aid and cardiopulmonary resuscitation (CPR). The National Safety Council's training network of nearly 10,000 instructors at over 4,000 sites worldwide has established the National Safety Council programs as the standard by which all others are judged.

In setting the standards, the National Safety Council has worked in close cooperation with hundreds of national and international organizations, thousands of corporations, thousands of leading educators, dozens of leading medical organizations, and hundreds of state and local governmental agencies. Their collective input has helped create programs that stand alone in quality. Consider just a few of the National Safety Council's current collaborations:

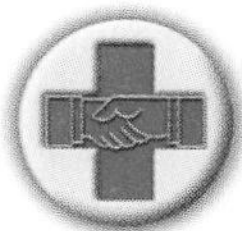

World's Leading Medical Organizations

The National Safety Council is currently working with both the American Academy of Orthopedic Surgeons (AAOS), Wilderness Medical Society (WMS), and the American Heart Association to help bring innovative, new training programs to the marketplace. The National Safety Council and the AAOS are developing a new First Responder program and the National Safety Council and the WMS are developing the first-of-its-kind wilderness first aid program.

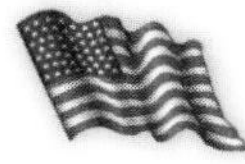

Spanning the Globe

Across the globe, from Boston to Bangkok, from Miami to Milan, from Seattle to Stockholm, people are trained with National Safety Council programs. National Safety Council first aid and CPR programs are already used in your area.

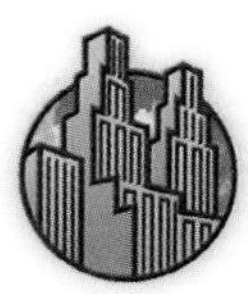

World's Leading Corporations

Thousands of corporations including Westinghouse, Exxon, General Motors, Ameritech, and U.S. West have selected many of the National Safety Council emergency care programs to train employees.

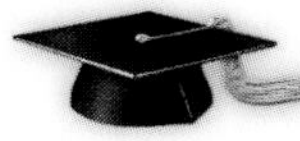

World's Leading Colleges and Universities

Hundreds of leading colleges and universities are working closely with the National Safety Council to fully develop and implement the Internet Initiative that will establish the National Safety Council as the leading online provider of emergency care programs.

Most importantly, in selecting the National Safety Council programs, you can feel confident that the programs are of the highest quality. You can rely on the National Safety Council. Founded in 1913, the National Safety Council is dedicated to protecting life, promoting health, and reducing accidental death. For nearly 90 years, the National Safety Council has been the world's leading authority on safety/injury education.

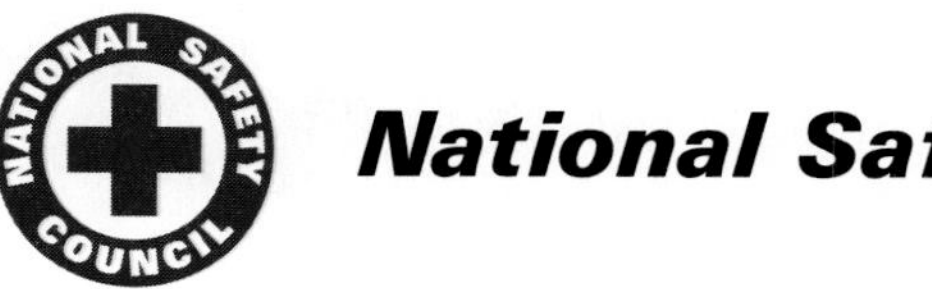

Table of Contents

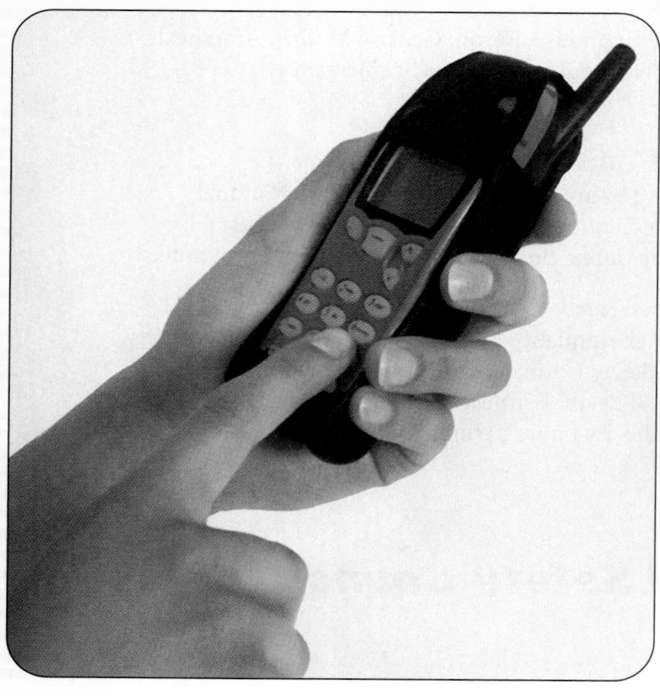

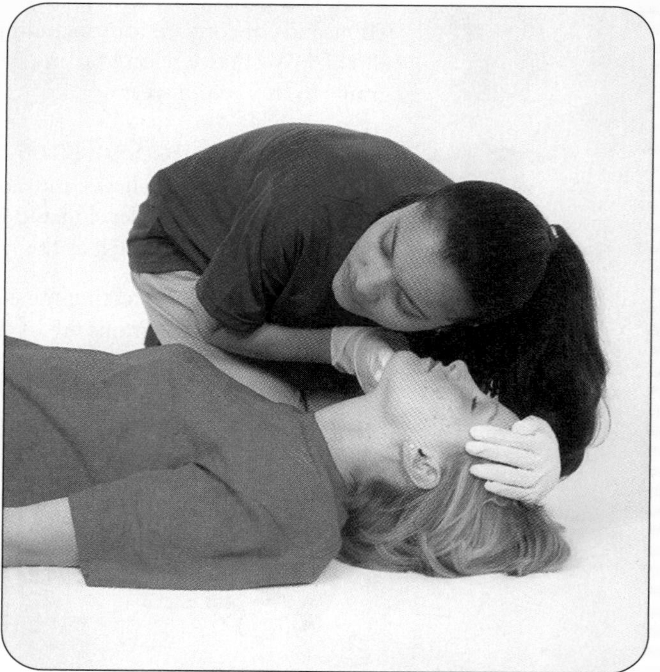

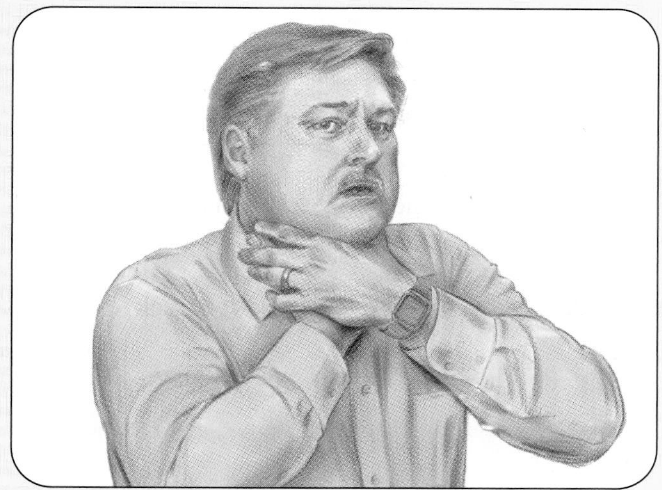

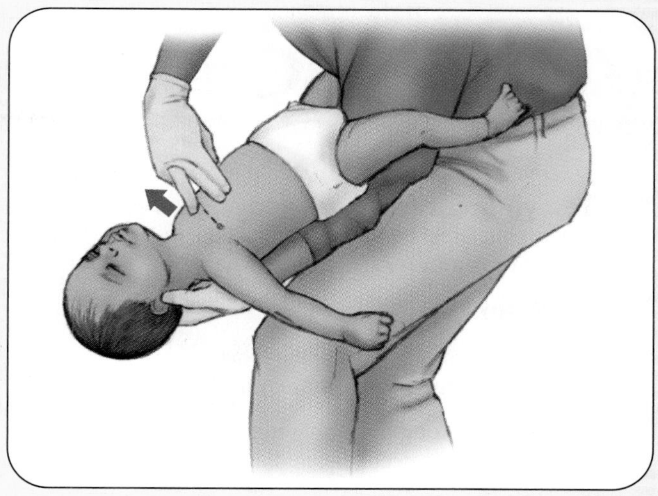

Your CPR IQ

Test your current knowledge. Read each question and place your answer in the "Pre-check" column. After reading this manual and completing your course, read the questions again and place your answers in the "Post-check" column. Compare your answers and see what you have learned.

Question	Pre-check			Post-check		
1. Most communities use 9-1-1 as their emergency telephone number.	T	F	Uncertain	T	F	Uncertain
2. Someone coughing forcefully is likely choking and needs immediately help.	T	F	Uncertain	T	F	Uncertain
3. Unresponsive, breathing victims should be placed on their side.	T	F	Uncertain	T	F	Uncertain
4. Adult CPR requires the rescuer to give 10 chest compressions and 1 rescue breath	T	F	Uncertain	T	F	Uncertain
5. Rescue breathing should be given to any unresponsive, non-breathing victim.	T	F	Uncertain	T	F	Uncertain
6. Open a victim's airway by tilting the head back and lifting the chin.	T	F	Uncertain	T	F	Uncertain
7. CPR should be performed on a firm, flat surface.	T	F	Uncertain	T	F	Uncertain
8. The procedures for child and infant CPR are the same as those for an adult.	T	F	Uncertain	T	F	Uncertain
9. Chest pain is one of the most frequent signals of a heart attack.	T	F	Uncertain	T	F	Uncertain
10. A sudden, severe headache and abnormal speech can be signals of a stroke	T	F	Uncertain	T	F	Uncertain

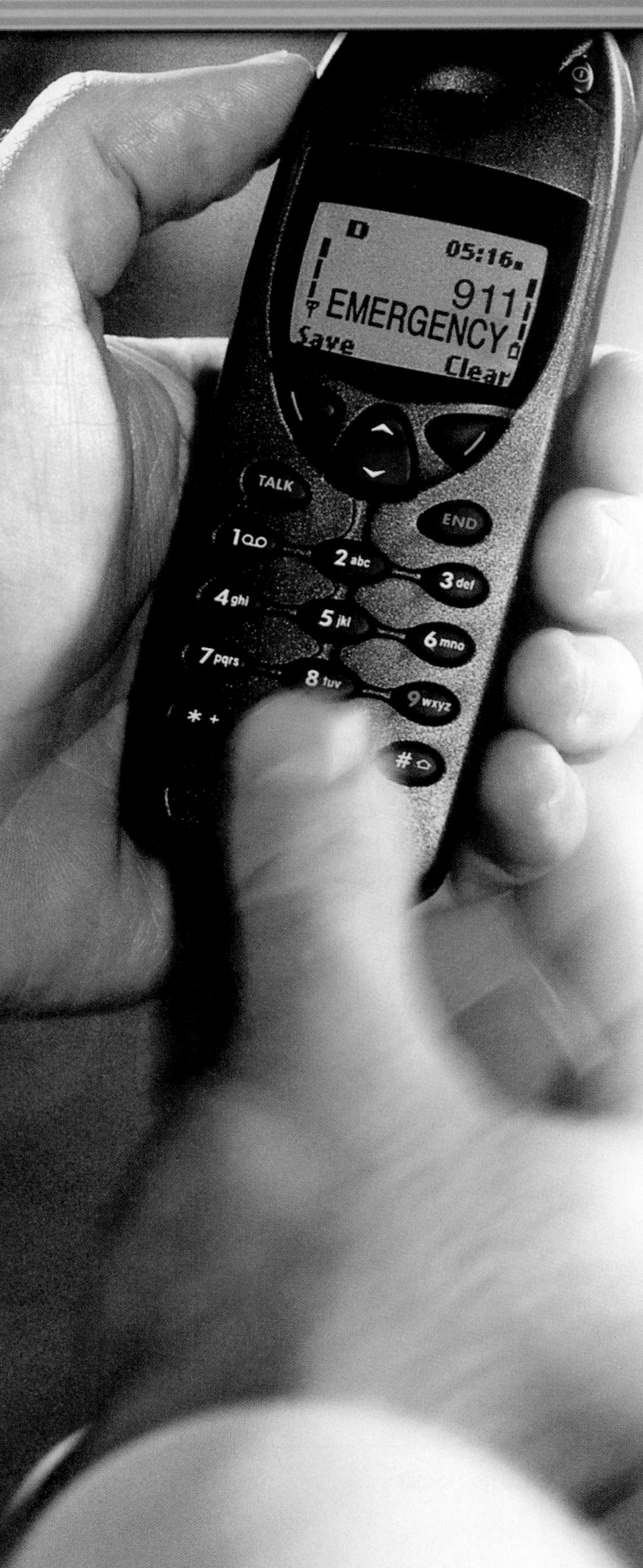

Chapter 1

Action at an Emergency

Bystander Intervention

Bystanders are a vital link between the emergency medical service (EMS) and the victim. In order to give a victim the best chance for survival, a bystander must quickly and reliably recognize the emergency and decide to help.

Everyone will at some time have to make a decision whether to help another person. A quick decision to get involved at the time of an emergency is unlikely to occur unless the bystander has considered the possibility of helping in advance. The most important time to make the decision to help is before you encounter an emergency.

Deciding to help is an attitude about helping people in emergencies and about one's competence to deal with emergencies.

Recognize the Emergency

To help in an emergency, the bystander has to notice that something is wrong—usually a person's appearance or behavior or the surroundings suggesting something unusual has happened.

Decide to Help

At some time, everyone will have to decide whether to help another person. Making a quick decision to get involved at the time of an emergency is unlikely to occur unless the bystander has previously considered the possibility of helping. Thus, **the most important time to make the decision to help is *before* you ever encounter an emergency.**

Deciding to help is an attitude about people, about emergencies, and about one's ability to deal with emergencies. It is an attitude that takes time to develop and is affected by a number of factors.

Call EMS, If Needed

People often make inappropriate decisions regarding calling EMS personnel. They delay calling for an ambulance until they are absolutely sure that an emergency exists, or they elect to bypass EMS personnel and transport the victim to medical care in a private vehicle. Such actions can present significant dangers to victims. Fortunately, most injuries and sudden illnesses that you will render care for will not require the need for advanced medical care—only first aid.

Assess the Victim

The bystander must decide if life-threatening conditions exist and what kind of help a victim needs immediately.

Provide Care

Often the most critical life-support measures are effective only if started immediately by the nearest available person. That person usually will be a layperson—a bystander.

Post-Care Reactions

After giving care for serious conditions, rescuers can feel an emotional "letdown," which is frequently overlooked. Discussing your feelings, fears, and reactions following the event can help prevent later emotional problems. You can talk to a trusted friend, a mental health professional, or a member of the clergy. Bringing out your feelings quickly helps to relieve personal anxieties and stress.

Scene Survey

If you are at the scene of an emergency situation, do a quick survey of the scene that includes looking for three things: (1) hazards that could be dangerous to you, the victim(s), or bystanders; (2) the cause (mechanism) of the injury or illness; and (3) the number of victims. This survey should only take a few seconds.

Seek Medical Attention

Knowing when to call for an ambulance is important. To know when to call, you must be able to tell the difference between a minor injury or illness and a life-threatening one. For example, upper abdominal pain can be as minor as indigestion or as severe as a heart attack needing prompt medical care. Wheezing may be related to a person's asthma, for which the person can use his or her prescribed inhaler for quick relief, or it can be as serious as a severe allergic reaction from a bee sting.

Not every cut needs stitches, nor does every burn require medical attention. It is, however, always best to err on the side of caution.

According to the American College of Emergency Physicians (ACEP), if the answer to any of the following questions is yes, or if you are unsure, call 9-1-1 or your local emergency number (if other from 9-1-1) for help.

- Is the victim's condition life-threatening?
- Could the condition get worse and become life-threatening on the way to the hospital?
- Does the victim need the skills or equipment of emergency medical technicians or paramedics?
- Would distance or traffic conditions cause a delay in getting to the hospital?

When a serious situation occurs, call EMS (9-1-1 in most communities) *first.* Do *not* call your doctor, the hospital, a friend, relatives, or neighbors for help before you call EMS. Calling anyone else first only wastes time.

How to Call EMS

To receive emergency assistance of every kind in most communities, you simply phone 9-1-1 (▼**Figure 1**). Check to see if this is true in your community. Emergency telephone numbers usually are listed on the inside front cover of telephone directories. Keep these numbers near or on every telephone. Call "0" (the operator) if you do not know the emergency number.

When you call EMS, the dispatcher will often ask for the following information. Speak slowly and clearly when you provide this information.

1. Your name and the phone number you are calling from. This prevents false calls and allows a dispatch center to call back if disconnected or for additional information if needed.
2. The victim's location. Give the address, names of intersecting roads, and other landmarks, if possible. Also, tell the specific location of the victim (eg, "in the basement").
3. What happened. State the nature of the emergency (eg, "My husband fell off a ladder and is not moving.").

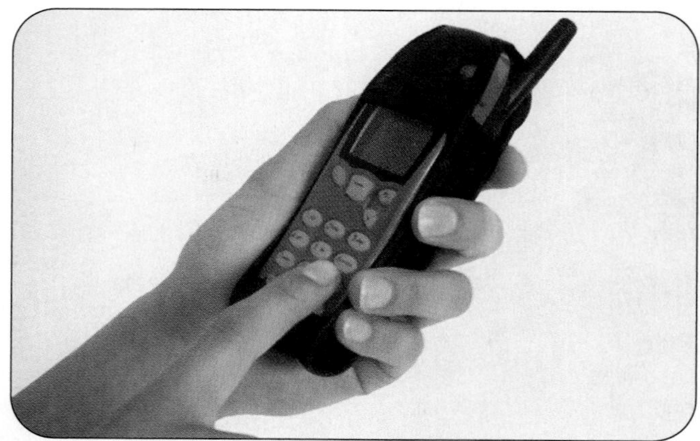

Figure 1 Call the local emergency number, 9-1-1, in most communities.

4. Number of persons needing help and any special conditions.
5. Victim's condition (eg, "My husband's head is bleeding.") and any first aid you have provided (such as pressing on the site of the bleeding).

Do *not* hang up the phone unless the dispatcher instructs you to do so. Enhanced 9-1-1 systems can track a call, but some communities lack this technology or are still using a seven-digit emergency number. Since cell phones can not be tracked through enhanced 9-1-1, it is important that the number be provided to the dispatcher and that all information is conveyed. Also, the EMS dispatcher may tell you how best to care for the victim. If you send someone else to call, have the person report back to you so you can be sure the call was made.

Disease Precautions

The risk of infectious diseases, can range from mild to life threatening. The risk of getting a disease from a victim is very low. But just the same, first aiders should know how to protect themselves against diseases carried by the blood and air. Precautionary measures help protect against infection from viruses and bacteria.

Bloodborne Disease

Some diseases are caused by microorganisms that are "borne" (carried) in a person's bloodstream. Contact with blood infected with such microorganisms may cause infection. Of the many blood-borne pathogens, three pose significant health threats to first aiders: hepatitis B virus (HBV), hepatitis C virus (HCV), and human immunodeficiency virus (HIV).

Hepatitis B

Hepatitis is a viral infection of the liver. Types A, B, and C are seen most often. Each is caused by a different virus.

A vaccine for hepatitis B is available and recommended for all infants and for adults who may have contact with carriers of the disease or with blood. Medical and laboratory workers, police, intravenous drug users, people with multiple sexual partners, and those living with someone who has a lifelong infection are at high risk of hepatitis B (and hepatitis C as well). Vaccination is the best defense against HBV. There is no chance of developing hepatitis B from the vaccine. Federal laws require employers to offer a series of three vaccine injections free to all employees who may be at risk of exposure.

Without vaccination shots, exposure to hepatitis B may produce symptoms within two weeks to six months after the exposure. People with hepatitis B infection may be symptom free, but that does *not* mean they are not contagious. These people may infect others who are exposed to their blood. Symptoms of hepatitis B resemble those of the flu and include fatigue, nausea, loss of appetite, stomach pain, and perhaps a yellowing of the skin.

Hepatitis B starts as an inflammation of the liver and usually lasts one to two months. In a few people, the infection is very serious, and in some, mild infection continues for life. The virus may stay in the liver and can lead to severe damage (cirrhosis) and liver cancer. Medical treatment that begins immediately after exposure may prevent the infection from developing.

Hepatitis C

Hepatitis C is caused by a different virus from HBV, but both diseases have a great deal in common. Like hepatitis B, hepatitis C affects the liver and can lead to long-term liver disease and liver cancer. Hepatitis C varies in severity and there may not be any symptoms at the time of infection. Currently, there is no vaccine or effective treatment for hepatitis C.

HIV

A person infected with HIV can infect others, and HIV-infected persons almost always develop acquired immunodeficiency syndrome (AIDS), which interferes with the body's ability to fight off other diseases. No vaccine is available to prevent HIV infection, which eventually proves fatal. The best defense against AIDS is to avoid becoming infected.

Protection

In most cases, you can control the risk of exposure to bloodborne pathogens by wearing the proper Personal Protective Equipment (PPE) and by following some simple procedures.

Personal Protective Equipment (PPE)

Personal protective equipment (PPE) prevents an organism from entering the body. The most common type of protection is when a rescuer uses medical exam gloves. The Food and Drug Administration (FDA), the Centers for Disease Control and Prevention (CDC), and the Occupational Safety and Health Administration (OSHA) have stated that vinyl and latex medical exam gloves are equally protective. Some rescuers are allergic to latex, and should wear vinyl or Nitrile gloves. All first aid kits should have several pairs of medical exam gloves (►Figure 2).

Protective eyewear and a standard surgical mask may be necessary at some emergencies; rescuers ordinarily will not have or need such equipment.

Mouth-to-barrier devices are available for rescue breathing and cardiopulmonary resuscitation (CPR). There are few documented cases of disease transmission to a rescuer as a result of performing unprotected CPR

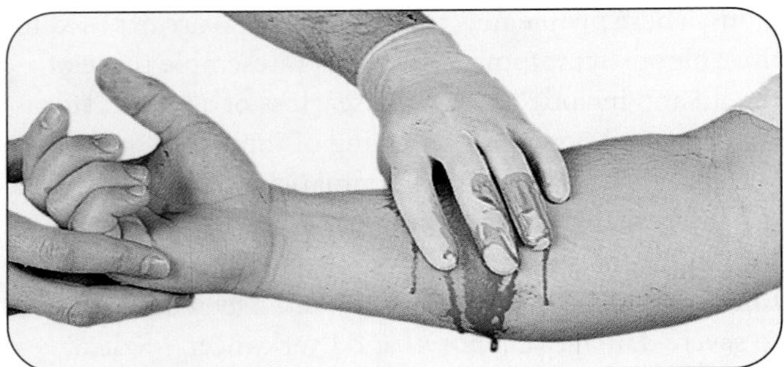

Figure 2 Whenever possible, use gloves as a barrier.

on an infected victim. Nevertheless, a mouth-to-barrier device should be used whenever possible ▼Figure 3.

Universal Precautions and Body Substance Isolation Techniques

Individuals infected with HBV or HIV may not show symptoms and may not even know they are infectious. For that reason, all human blood and body fluids should be considered infectious, and precautions should be taken to avoid contact. The *body substance isolation* (BSI) technique assumes that *any* body fluid is a possible risk. EMS personnel routinely follow BSI procedures, even if blood or body fluids are not visible.

OSHA requires any company with employees who are expected to give first aid in an emergency to follow *universal precautions,* which assume that *all* blood and *certain* body fluids pose a risk for transmission of HBV and HIV. OSHA defines an employee who assists another with a nosebleed or a cut as a "Good Samaritan." Such acts, however, are not considered occupational exposure unless the employee who provided the assistance is a member of a first aid team or is designated or expected to render first aid as part of his or her job. In essence, OSHA's requirement excludes unassigned employees who perform unanticipated first aid.

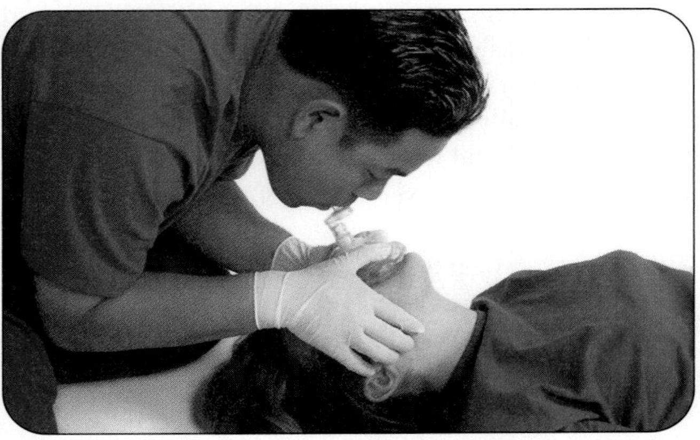

Figure 3 Face mask, one-way valve

Whenever there is a chance that you could be exposed to bloodborne pathogens, your employer must provide appropriate PPE, which might include eye protection, medical exam gloves, gowns, and masks. The PPE must be accessible, and your employer must provide training to help you choose the right PPE for your work.

While EMS personnel follow BSI procedures and OSHA requires designated worksite first aiders to follow universal precautions, what should a typical first aider do? It makes sense for first aiders to follow BSI procedures and assume that *all* blood and body fluids are infectious and follow appropriate protective measures.

Coping with Emergencies

When an incident occurs, you can protect yourself and others against bloodborne pathogens by following these steps:

1. Use appropriate PPE, such as gloves, and a resuscitation mask.
2. If you have been trained in the correct procedures, use absorbent barriers to soak up blood or other infectious materials.
3. Clean the spill area with an appropriate disinfecting solution, such as diluted bleach.
4. Discard contaminated materials in an appropriate waste disposal container.

If you have been exposed to blood or body fluids:

1. Use soap and water to wash the parts of your body that have been contaminated.
2. Report the incident to your supervisor, if the exposure happens while at work. Otherwise, contact your personal physician. Early action can prevent the development of hepatitis B and enable affected workers to track potential HIV infection.

The best protection against bloodborne disease is to use the safeguards described here. By following these guidelines, you can decrease your chance of contracting bloodborne illnesses.

Airborne Disease

Infective organisms such as bacteria or viruses that are introduced into the air by coughing or sneezing are said to be "airborne." Droplets of mucus that carry those bacteria or viruses can then be inhaled by other individuals. The rate of tuberculosis (TB) has increased recently and is receiving much attention. TB, caused by bacteria, sometimes settles in the lungs and can be fatal. In most cases, a first aider will not know that a victim has TB. Assume that any person with a cough, especially one who is in a nursing home or a shelter, may have TB. Other symptoms include fatigue, weight loss, chest pain, and coughing up blood. If a surgical mask is available, wear it or wrap a handkerchief over your nose and mouth.

Legal Considerations

Fear of lawsuits has made some people reluctant about getting involved at emergency scenes. Rescuers, however, are rarely sued; those who are usually receive a favorable ruling from courts.

Consent

Before giving care, a rescuer must have the victim's consent (permission). Touching another person without his or her permission or consent is unlawful (known as battery) and could be grounds for a lawsuit. Likewise, giving care without the victim's consent is unlawful.

Expressed Consent

Consent must be obtained from every conscious, mentally competent (able to make a rational decision) person of legal age. Tell the victim your name and that you have training, and explain what you will be doing. Permission from the victim may be expressed either with words or with a nod of the head.

Implied Consent

Implied consent involves an unresponsive victim in a life-threatening condition. It is assumed or "implied" that an unresponsive victim would consent to lifesaving help. When a child is in a life-threatening situation, and the parent or legal guardian is not available for consent, first aid should be given based on implied consent. Do not withhold care from a minor just to obtain parental or guardian permission.

Abandonment

Abandonment means leaving a victim after starting to give help without ensuring someone else will continue the care at the same level or higher. Once you have started providing care, you must not leave a victim who still needs first aid until another competent and trained person takes responsibility for the victim.

Negligence

Negligence means not following accepted standards of care and causing injury to the victim. Negligence involves:

1. Having a duty to act
2. Breaching that duty (by giving substandard care)
3. Causing injury and damages

Duty to Act

No one is required to render care when no legal duty exists. Duty to act may occur in the following situations:

- *When your employment requires it.* If your employer designates you as responsible for rendering care to meet OSHA (Occupational Safety and Health Administration) requirements and you are called to an injury scene, you have a duty to act. Examples of occupations with job descriptions that include a duty to act include law enforcement officers, park rangers, athletic trainers, lifeguards, and teachers.
- *When a pre-existing responsibility exists.* You may have a pre-existing relationship with other persons that demands you be responsible for them, which means you must give first aid if they need it. Examples include a parent for a child, or a driver for a passenger.

Duty to act means following guidelines for standards of care. Standards of care ensure quality care and protection for injured or suddenly ill victims.

Breach of Duty

Generally, a rescuer breaches (breaks) his or her duty to a victim by failing to provide the type of care that would be provided by a person having the same or similar training. One's duty can be breached by acts of omission or acts of commission. An *act of omission* is the failure to do what a reasonably prudent person with the same or similar training would do in the same or similar circumstances. An *act of commission* is doing something that a reasonably prudent person would *not* do under the same or similar circumstances.

Injury and Damages Inflicted

Injury or damages must have resulted from a breach of duty. In addition to physical damage, injury and damage can include physical pain and suffering, mental anguish, medical expenses, and sometimes loss of earnings and earning capacity.

Good Samaritan Laws

In most emergencies, you are not legally required to give care. To encourage people to assist others needing help, Good Samaritan laws grant immunity against lawsuits. Although laws vary from state to state, Good Samaritan immunity generally applies only when the rescuer is (1) acting during an emergency, (2) acting in good faith, which means he or she has good intentions, (3) acting without compensation, and (4) not guilty of any malicious misconduct or gross negligence toward the victim (deviating from all rational first aid guidelines).

Good Samaritan laws are not a substitute for competent care or for keeping within the scope of your training.

To find out about your state's Good Samaritan laws, ask for information at your local library or an attorney.

Learning Activities

Action at an Emergency

Directions: Circle Yes if you agree with the statement, and circle No if you disagree.

Yes No **1.** In most locations an ambulance can arrive within minutes. This quick response means that most people do not need to learn CPR.

Yes No **2.** Good Samaritan laws help protect lay rescuers when they provide help in an emergency.

Yes No **3.** A scene survey should be done before providing care.

Yes No **4.** Most communities use the 9-1-1 telephone number for emergencies.

Yes No **5.** If you ask a person if you can help, and she says "No," you can ignore her and proceed to provide care.

Chapter 2

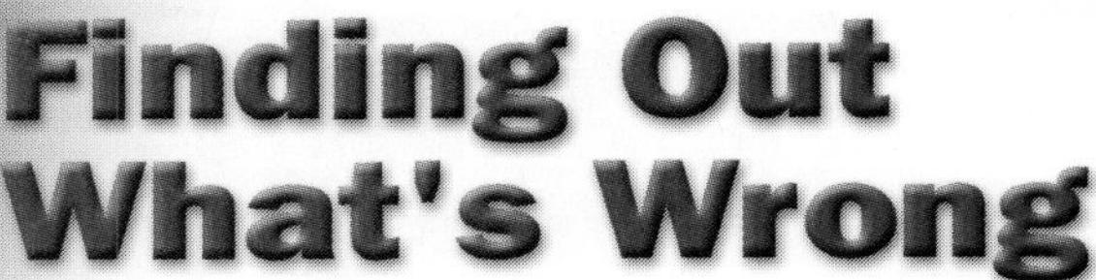

Finding Out What's Wrong

Victim Assessment

Victim assessment is an important skill. It requires an understanding of each assessment step as well as decision-making skills.

Every time you encounter a victim, first check out the scene. The scene survey determines the safety of the scene, the victim's cause of injury or nature of illness, and the number of victims. Without a scene survey, a potentially dangerous situation could result in further injury to the victim or to you and others.

The scene survey is followed by the initial victim assessment. During the initial victim assessment, you identify and correct immediate life-threatening conditions involving problems with the victim's airway, breathing, and circulation (the ABCs). Victims with immediate life-threatening conditions can die within minutes unless their problems are quickly recognized and corrected. Determining the type of injury or illness is also part of the initial assessment.

Initial Assessment

The goal of the initial assessment is to determine whether there are life-threatening problems that require quick care (►**Skill Scan**). This assessment involves evaluating the victim's airway (A), breathing (B), and circulation (C). The following step-by-step initial assessment should not be changed. It takes less than a minute to complete, unless care is required at any point. By the end of the initial assessment, the victim's problem will most likely be identified as being an injury or an illness.

Begin the initial assessment with a check for responsiveness. If there is a possibility of a spinal injury, have another person hold the victim's head to minimize movement and avoid causing further damage (►**Figure 1**).

Check for responsiveness by speaking to the victim. If the person can talk, breathing and heartbeat are present. If the victim does not respond, tap his or her shoulder and ask, "Are you okay?" If there is no response, consider the victim as being unresponsive.

Skill Scan Initial Assessment

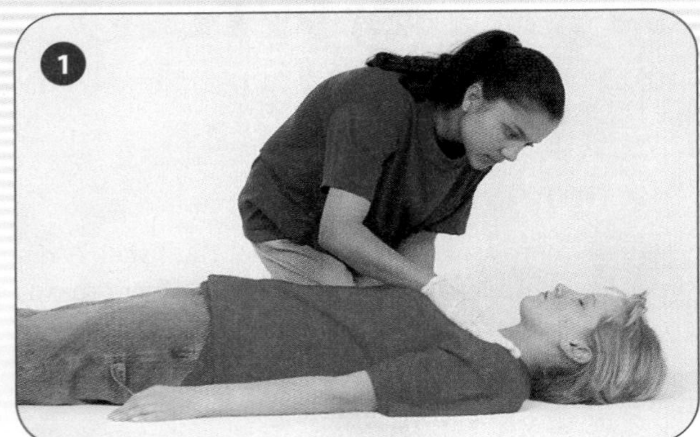

1. Responsive? Tap and shout.

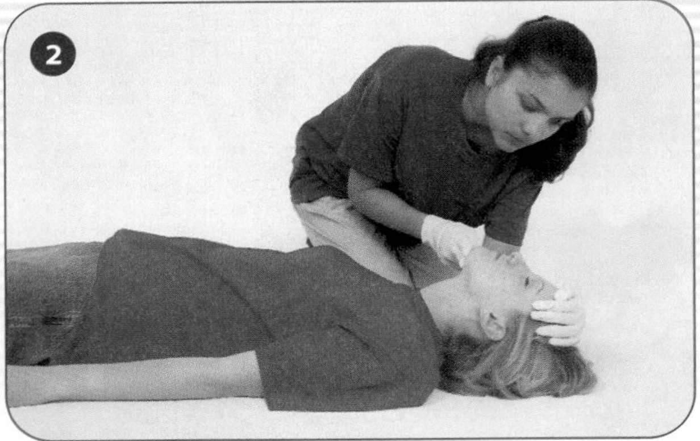

2. A = Airway open? Head-tilt/chin-lift.

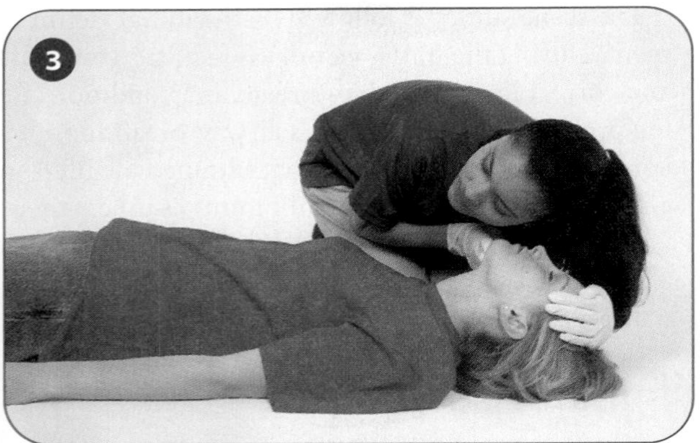

3. B = Breathing? Look, listen, and feel.

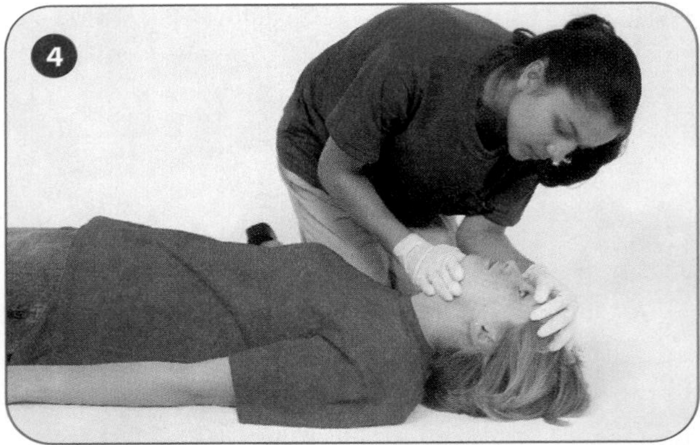

4. C = Circulation? Check for signs of circulation.

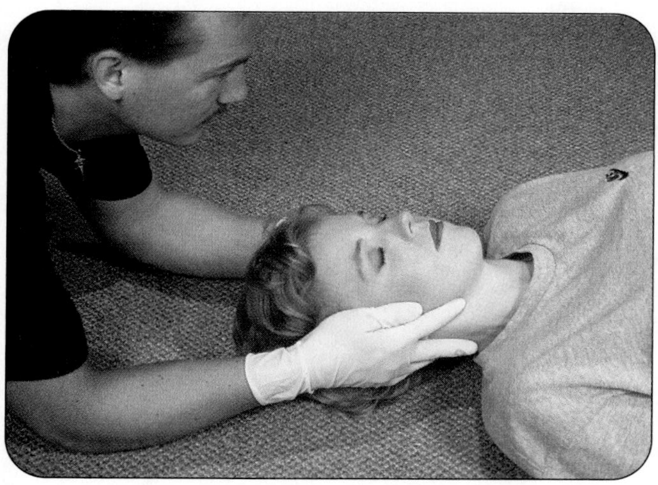

Figure 1 Immobilizing the head with the hands

Immediate Threats to Life

A: Airway

The airway must be open for breathing. If the victim is speaking or crying, the airway is open. If a responsive victim cannot talk, cry, or cough forcefully, the airway is probably obstructed and must be checked and cleared. In this case, abdominal thrusts (Heimlich maneuver) can be given to clear an obstructed airway in a responsive adult victim.

In an unresponsive victim lying face up, the most common airway obstruction is the tongue. Snoring is evidence of this. If there is no suspected spinal injury, use the head-tilt/chin-lift method to open the airway. If a spinal cord injury is likely, use the jaw-thrust method without head tilt to prevent further injury.

Once the victim's airway is clear of obstruction, the initial assessment can continue.

B: Breathing

A breathing rate between 12 and 20 times per minute is normal for adults. Victims who are having difficulty moving air and who are breathing less than eight times per minute or more than 24 times per minute need care. Note any breathing difficulties or unusual breathing sounds such as wheezing, crowing, gurgling, or snoring. This step primarily focuses upon whether or not the victim is breathing and obvious breathing difficulties rather than the breathing rate.

Check for breathing in an unresponsive victim after opening the airway. Watch for the victim's chest to rise and fall as you place your ear next to the victim's mouth. "Look, listen, and feel" for about 10 seconds to check for breathing. If the victim is not breathing, keep the airway open and breathe two slow rescue breaths into the victim. Rescue breathing is discussed in detail in the next chapter.

C: Circulation

After checking and correcting any airway and breathing problems, check the victim's circulation.This can be done by checking the signs of circulation—breathing, coughing, movement and noting skin condition, and pulse. If signs of circulation are absent, begin cardiopulmonary resuscitation (CPR) until a defibrillator is available. CPR is discussed in detail in the next chapter. Defibrillation is discussed in Appendix B.

Severe Bleeding Check for severe bleeding by looking over the victim's entire body for blood (blood-soaked clothing or blood pooling on the floor or the ground). Controlling bleeding requires the application of direct pressure or a pressure bandage.

Skin Condition A quick check of the victim's skin can also provide information about circulatory status. Check skin temperature, color, and condition (eg, moist, dry). Skin color, especially in light-skinned people, reflects the circulation under the skin as well as oxygen status. In darkly pigmented people, changes might not be readily apparent but can be assessed by the appearance of the nail beds, the inside of the mouth, and the inner eyelids. When the skin's blood vessels constrict or circulation slows, or stops, the skin becomes cool and pale or cyanotic (blue-gray color). When the skin's blood vessels dilate or blood flow increases, the skin becomes warm.

Learning Activities

Finding Out What is Wrong

Directions: Circle Yes if you agree with the statement, and circle No if you disagree.

Yes No **1.** The purpose of the initial assessment is to find life-threatening conditions.

Yes No **2.** The initial assessment begins with a check for signs of circulation.

Yes No **3.** The airway can be opened using the head-tilt/chin-lift technique.

Yes No **4.** A person who is not breathing needs rescue breathing.

Yes No **5.** A person without signs of circulation needs CPR.

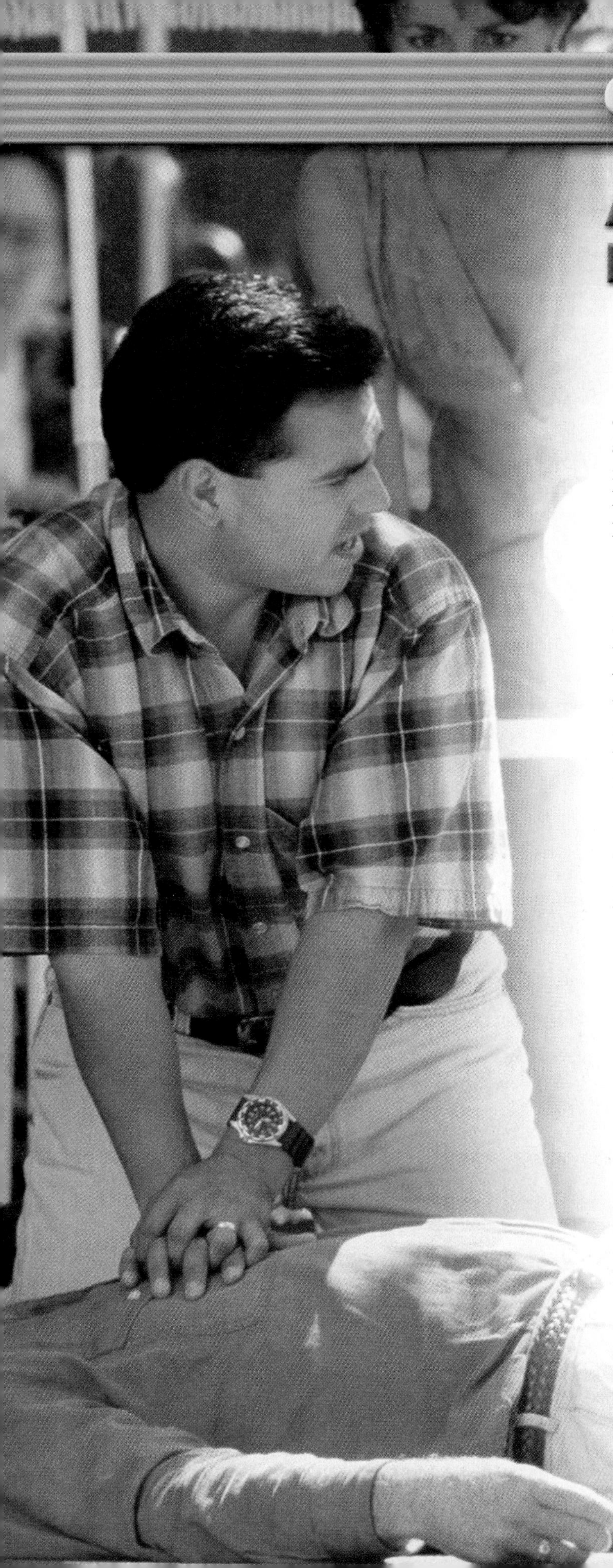

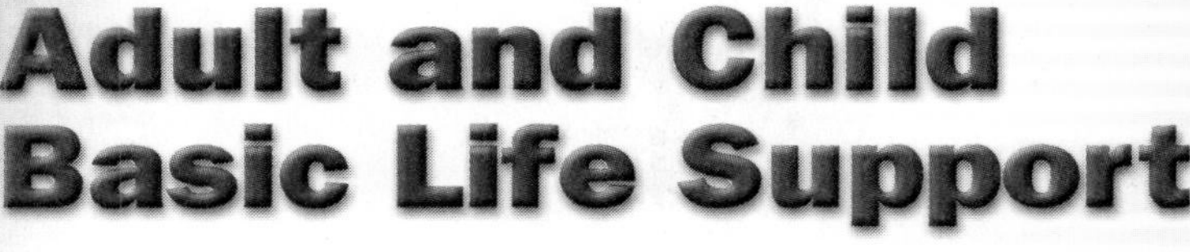

Adult and Child Basic Life Support

Heart attacks causing heart stoppage (cardiac arrest) are the most prominent cause of death in North America. In addition, drowning, suffocation, electrocution, and drug intoxication cause cardiac arrest. Many deaths could be prevented if the victims receive early CPR, early automated external defibrillation (AED), and early advanced care by trained EMS professionals (►Figure 1).

Rescue Breathing

For the unresponsive breathing victim, place him or her in the recovery position (►Figure 2). For the non-breathing victim, rescue breathing must be started immediately. Roll the victim onto his or her back (►Figure 3). If the victim is not breathing, perform rescue breathing by using one of the following methods: mouth-to-mouth, mouth-to-nose, mouth-to-stoma, or mouth-to-barrier device.

Mouth-to-Mouth Method

The mouth-to-mouth method of rescue breathing is a simple, quick, and effective method for an emergency situation. With the airway open, pinch the nose shut, take a breath, and breathe into the victim with slow breaths. Each breath should be just enough to make the chest rise.

Do not remove a victim's dentures unless they interfere with rescue breathing. Even loose dentures give form and shape to the victim's mouth.

Mouth-to-Nose Method

Although mouth-to-mouth breathing is successful in the majority of cases, certain complications may necessitate mouth-to-nose rescue breathing. For example, if you cannot open the victim's mouth, their teeth are clenched together, you cannot make a good seal around the victim's mouth, the victim's mouth is severely injured, or the victim's mouth is too large or has no teeth.

The mouth-to-nose technique is performed like mouth-to-mouth breathing, except that you force your exhaled breath through the victim's nose while holding his or her mouth closed with one hand pushing up on the chin. The victim's mouth then must be held open so any nasal obstruction does not impede exhalation of air from the victim's lungs.

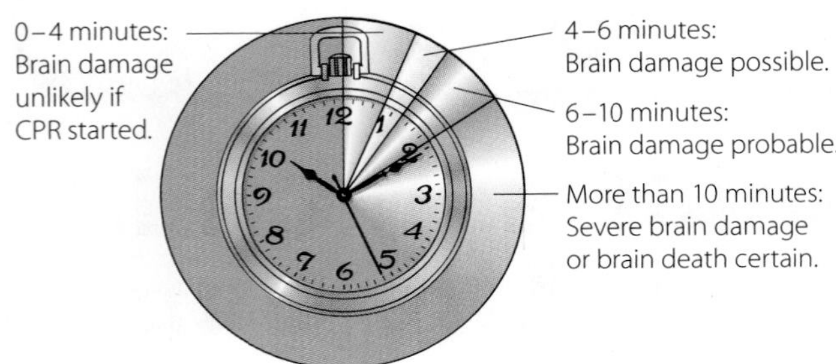
0–4 minutes:
Brain damage
unlikely if
CPR started.
4–6 minutes:
Brain damage possible.
6–10 minutes:
Brain damage probable.
More than 10 minutes:
Severe brain damage
or brain death certain.

Figure 1 Start resuscitation efforts at once. Brain damage occurs without oxygen.

Mouth-to-Stoma Method

Cancer and other diseases of the vocal cords may make surgical removal of the larynx necessary. People who have had this surgery breathe through a small permanent opening in the lower part of the neck called a *stoma*, which is surgically made and joined to the trachea.

In mouth-to-stoma rescue breathing, the victim's mouth and nose must be closed during the delivery of breaths because the air can flow upward into the upper airway through the larynx as well as downward into the lungs. You can close the victim's mouth and nose with one hand. Determine breathing by looking at, listening to, and feeling the stoma. Keep the victim's head and neck level.

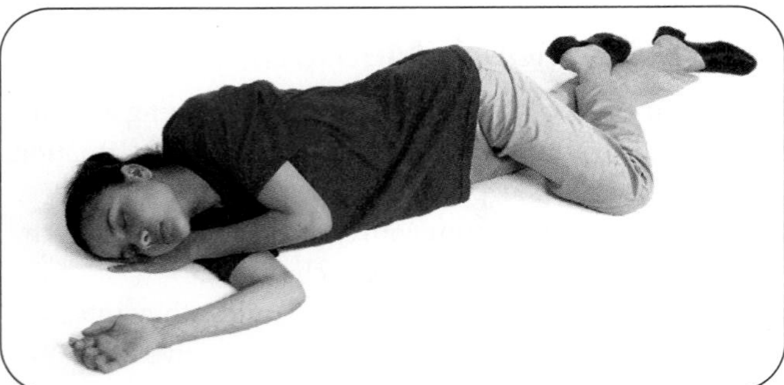

Figure 2 Recovery position. The hand supports the head. Chin tilted. Bent knee and arm give stability.

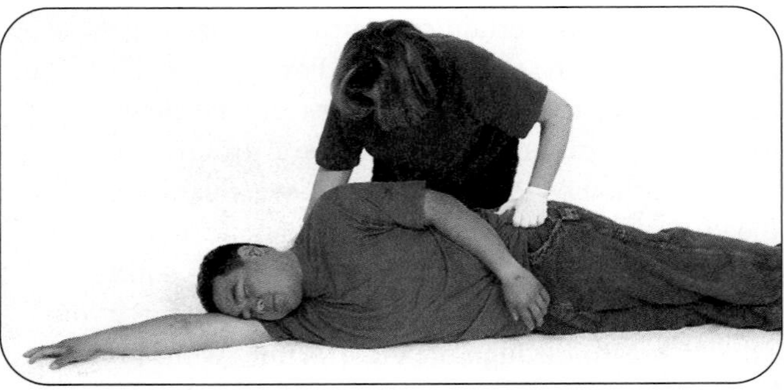

Figure 3 Support the head and neck with one hand. Firmly grip the clothing or edge of the hip with your other hand. Roll the victim over.

Gastric Distention

Rescue breathing can cause stomach or gastric distention more often in infants than in adults. Minimize this problem by limiting the breaths to the amount needed to make the chest rise. Avoid overinflating the lungs. Gastric distention can cause regurgitation and aspiration of stomach contents.

Mouth-to-Barrier Device

A mouth-to-barrier device is an apparatus that is placed over a victim's face as a safety precaution for the rescuer during rescue breathing (▼**Figure 4A–B**). There are two types of mouth-to-barrier devices:

- *Masks.* Resuscitation masks are clear, plastic devices that cover the victim's mouth and nose. They have a one-way valve so exhaled air from the victim does not enter the rescuer's mouth.
- *Face shields.* These clear plastic devices have a mouthpiece through which the rescuer breathes (►**Figure 5**). Some models have a short airway that is inserted into the victim's mouth over the tongue. They are smaller and less expensive than masks, but air can leak around the shield. Also, they cover only the victim's mouth, so the nose must be pinched.

After the barrier device is in place, the rescuer breathes through the device. The technique is performed like mouth-to-mouth breathing. See the skill sheets in this chapter for the steps for performing rescue breathing.

Airway Obstruction (Choking)

Recognizing Choking

A foreign body lodged in the airway may cause partial or complete airway obstruction. When a foreign body partially blocks the airway, either good or poor air exchange

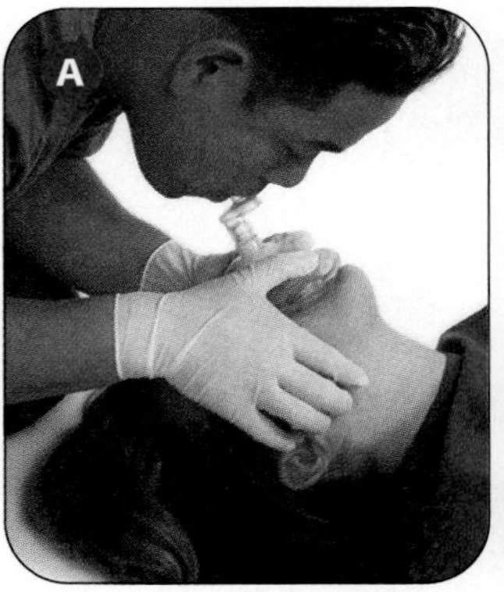
A

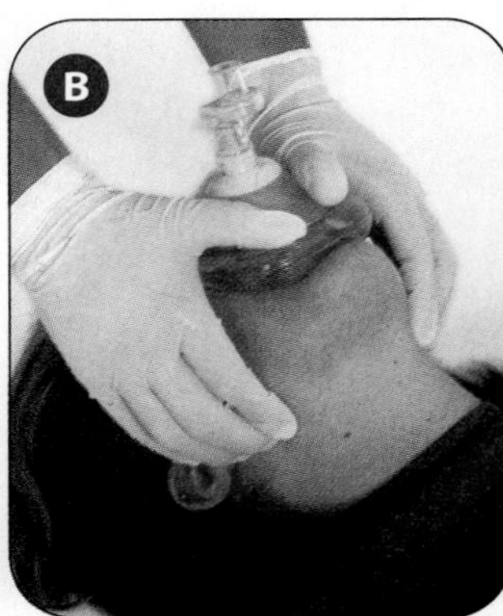
B

Figure 4A–B Mouth-to-barrier device—mask.

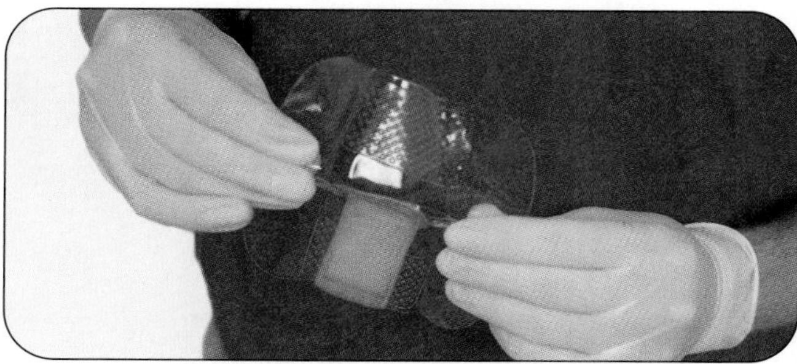

Figure 5 Face shield

may result. When good air exchange is present, the victim is able to make forceful coughing efforts in an attempt to relieve the obstruction. The victim should be permitted and encouraged to cough. Sometimes, however, a good air exchange may progress to a poor air exchange.

A choking victim who has poor air exchange has a weak and ineffective cough, and breathing becomes more difficult. The skin, the fingernail beds, and the inside of the mouth may appear bluish-gray in color. Each attempt to inhale is usually accompanied by a high-pitched noise. A partial airway obstruction with poor air exchange should be treated as if it were a complete airway blockage.

Complete airway obstruction in a responsive victim commonly occurs when the victim has been eating. Children and infants choke on all kinds of objects. Foods such as hot dogs, candy, peanuts, and grapes are major offenders because of their shape and consistencies. Nonfood choking deaths are caused by balloons, balls, marbles, toys, and coins. With complete airway obstruction, the victim is unable to speak, breathe, or cough. When asked, "Can you speak?" the victim is unable to respond verbally. Choking victims with complete foreign body obstruction of the airway may instinctively reach up and clutch their necks to communicate that they are choking. This motion is known as the distress signal for choking ►Figure 6. The victim becomes panicked and desperate and may appear pale in color. Because a complete obstruction prevents air from entering the lungs, oxygen deprivation occurs within a few minutes.

Complete airway obstruction in an unresponsive victim is usually the result of the tongue relaxing in the back of the mouth, restricting air movement. Simply positioning the airway can correct this problem. See the skill sheets in this chapter for the steps for clearing an airway obstruction.

Types of Upper Airway Obstruction

- *Tongue.* Unconsciousness produces relaxation of soft tissues, and the tongue can fall into the airway. "Swallowing one's tongue" is impossible, but the widespread belief that it can happen is explained by slippage of the relaxed tongue into the airway. The tongue is the most common cause of airway obstruction.
- *Foreign body.* The National Safety Council reports that more than 2,000 deaths occur in the United States each year because of foreign body airway obstruction. People, especially children, inhale all kinds of objects. Foods such as hotdogs, candy, peanuts, and grapes are major offenders because of their shapes and consistencies. Meat is the main cause of choking in adults. Balloons are the top cause of nonfood choking deaths in children, followed by balls, marbles, toys, and coins. Unconscious victims' airways also can be obstructed by a foreign body (eg, vomit, teeth).
- *Swelling.* Severe allergic reactions (anaphylaxis) and irritants (eg, smoke, chemicals) can cause swelling. Even a nonallergic person who is stung inside the throat by a bee, yellow jacket, or flying insect can experience swelling in the airway.
- *Spasm.* Water that is suddenly inhaled can cause a spasm in the throat. This happens in about 10 percent of all drownings. When such a spasm does not allow the lungs to fill with water, it is known as a "dry drowning."
- *Vomit.* Most people vomit when they are at or near death. Therefore, always expect vomit during CPR.

Care for Choking

Giving abdominal thrusts to a choking victim can dislodge the foreign body from the airway. To give abdominal thrusts to a choking victim, position yourself behind the victim. Place your arms around the victim's waist and form a fist with one hand. Place the thumb side of the fist with the knuckles up against the victim's abdomen slightly above the navel. With your other hand, grasp and hold your fist, then give quick upward and inward thrusts to the victim's abdomen ►Figure 7.

A conscious choking victim who is alone can self-administer abdominal thrusts. The victim places the thumb side of

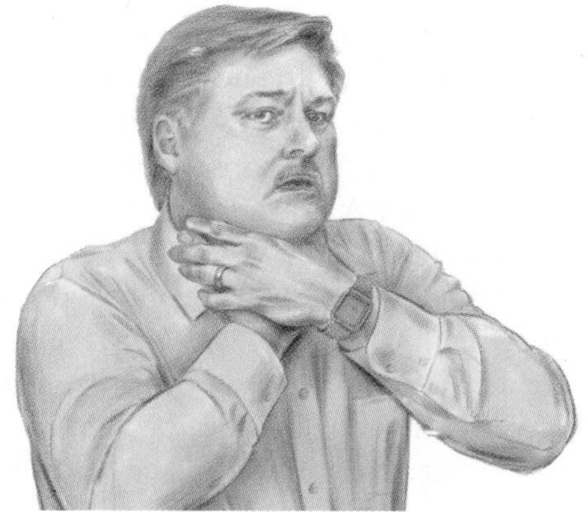

Figure 6 Universal sign of choking distress.

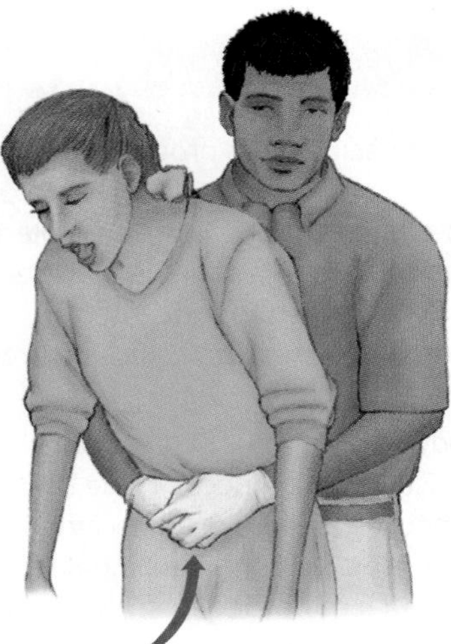

Figure 7 Abdominal thrust for a responsive victim.

a closed fist in the same position described above, covers the fist with the other hand, then gives inward, upward thrusts. Also, if a firm object such as a chair or table is available, the victim can lean over the back of the chair or a corner of the table, pressing the abdomen upward and inward.

If the choking victim is obese or in an advanced stage of pregnancy, give chest thrusts. Position yourself behind the victim and place the thumb side of a fist on the middle of the victim's sternum. Then thrust straight back. See the skill sheets in this chapter for the detailed steps for clearing an airway obstruction.

History of Resuscitation

Throughout the centuries, resuscitation attempts have included:

Unsuccessful methods:

- slapping a victim
- dousing a victim with hot or cold water
- whipping a victim with stinging nettles
- making loud noises
- building a fire on a victim's abdomen

Occasionally successful methods:

- rolling a drowned victim back and forth over a barrel
- throwing a victim across the back of a trotting horse
- blowing air into a victim with fireplace bellows
- pulling a victim's arms
- pressing a victim's back

The mouth-to-mouth breathing method (today known as rescue breathing) was sometimes reported prior to the 1950s. Since the 1950s, it has been the preferred method.

Medical researchers in 1960 discovered that compressing a victim's chest along with rescue breathing could help sustain life for a brief time period after the heart had stopped. At first, only physicians, nurses, and emergency medical aides were taught to perform the technique. In 1973, CPR began being taught to the public, not just to medically trained personnel.

The Heimlich maneuver (also known as abdominal thrusts) was first described by its developer, Dr. Henry J. Heimlich, in a 1974 medical journal.

Cardiopulmonary Resuscitation (CPR)

One of the leading causes of death for adults in the United States is sudden cardiac arrest, resulting in about 250,000 deaths each year.

Causes of Cardiac Arrest

Most sudden cardiac arrest victims have an electrical malfunction of the heart termed ventricular fibrillation. In ventricular fibrillation, the heart's electrical signals, which normally induce a coordinated heartbeat, suddenly become chaotic, and the heart's pumping function abruptly ceases. When the heart stops pumping blood, the victim immediately loses consciousness and is considered clinically dead. A heart in ventricular fibrillation quivers like a bowl of gelatin. When this occurs, the heart is not pumping blood and there are only about four minutes to correct this problem before irreversible brain damage occurs. Without intervention, the victim will become biologically (irreversibly) dead within minutes. When a person's heart stops beating, he or she needs CPR until a defibrillator is available. CPR is the process of giving rescue breaths and chest compressions to move oxygen throughout the victim's body.

Chest compressions are performed with 2 hands (adult) or 1 hand (child). The desired position on the chest is between the nipples, on the lower half of the sternum (►Figure 8). For chest compressions to be effective, the victim must be on a firm, flat surface. Refer to the skill sheets for detailed CPR procedures.

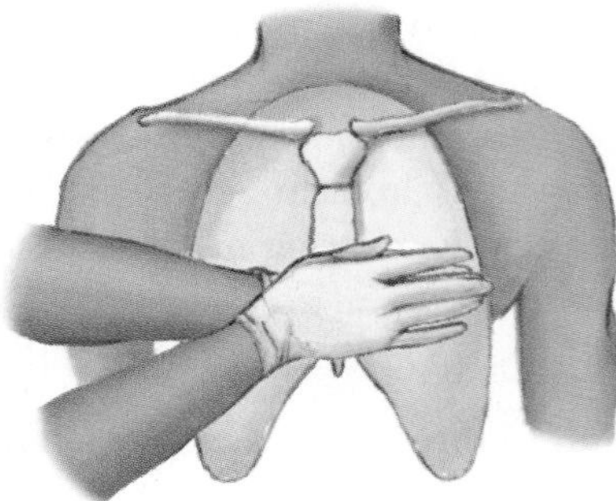

Figure 8 Proper hand placement for chest compressions.

BASIC LIFE SUPPORT

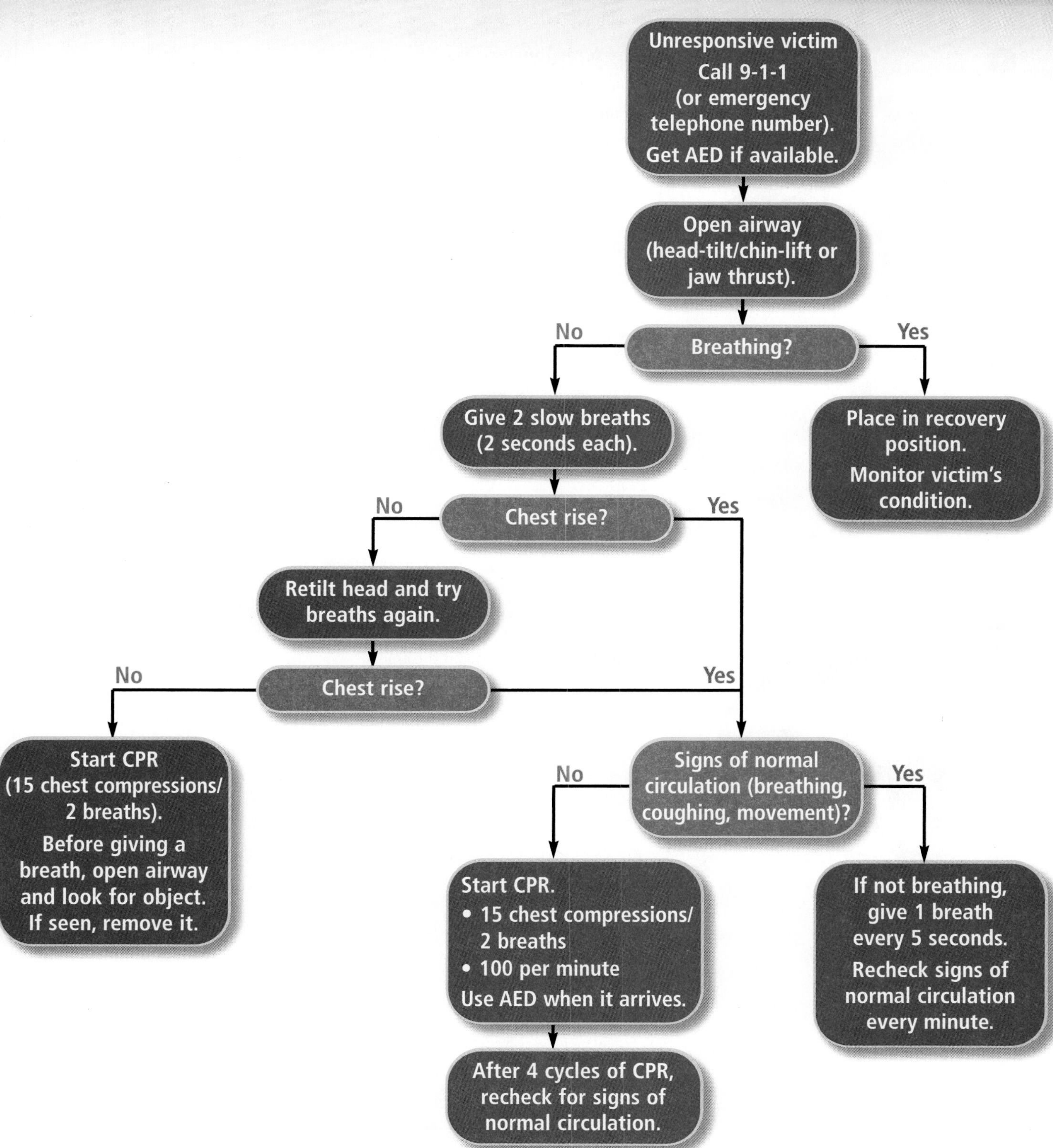

Unresponsive victim
Call 9-1-1
(or emergency telephone number).
Get AED if available.
Open airway
(head-tilt/chin-lift or jaw thrust).
Breathing?
No
Yes
Place in recovery position.
Monitor victim's condition.
Give 2 slow breaths
(2 seconds each).
Chest rise?
No
Yes
Retilt head and try breaths again.
Chest rise?
No
Yes
Start CPR
(15 chest compressions/ 2 breaths).
Before giving a breath, open airway and look for object. If seen, remove it.
Signs of normal circulation (breathing, coughing, movement)?
No
Yes
Start CPR.
• 15 chest compressions/ 2 breaths
• 100 per minute
Use AED when it arrives.
If not breathing, give 1 breath every 5 seconds.
Recheck signs of normal circulation every minute.
After 4 cycles of CPR, recheck for signs of normal circulation.

Basic Life Support
Adult and Child Rescue Breathing and CPR

If you see a motionless person . . .

1

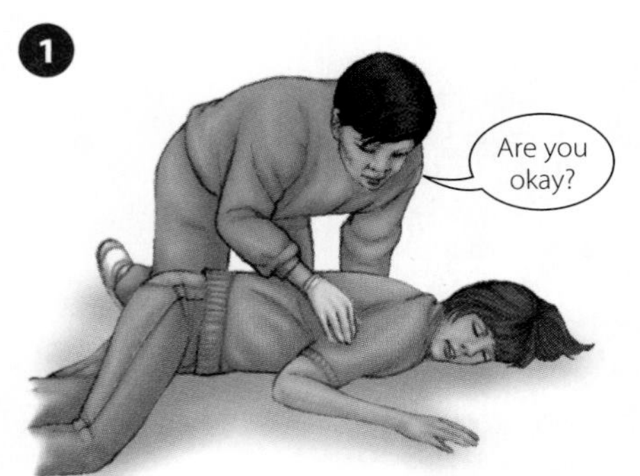

Check responsiveness
- Tap the victim and shout, "Are you okay?"
- If unresponsive, go to step #2.

2

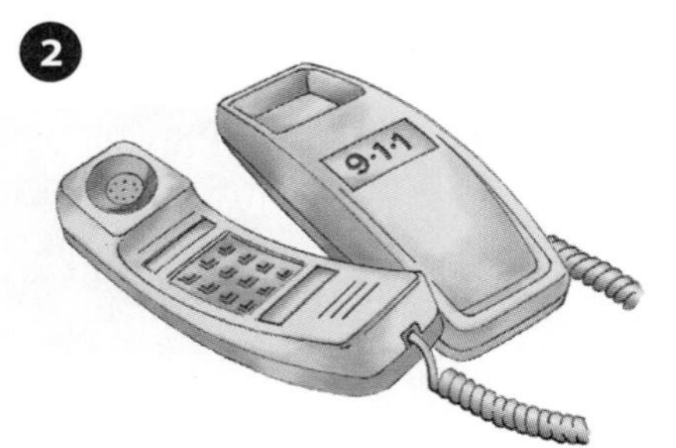

Call 9-1-1 or emergency telephone number
- If the victim is 8 years of age or older and an AED is available, get it.

3

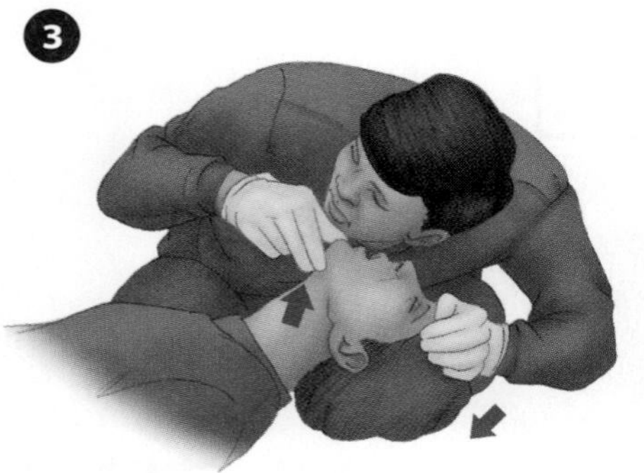

Open airway
- Tilt the head back and lift the chin.
- Remove any obvious obstructions.
- If you suspect a spinal injury, use jaw-thrust method without head-tilt.

Basic Life Support
Adult and Child Rescue Breathing and CPR

4a

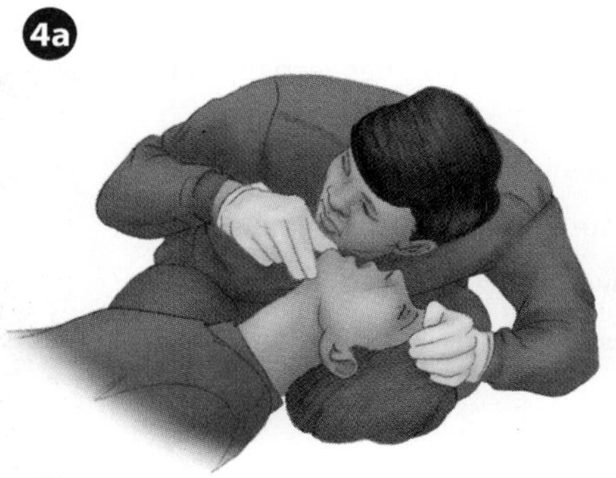

4b

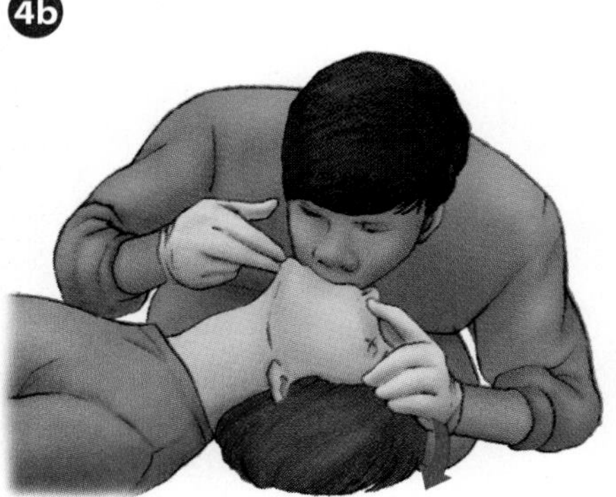

Check breathing (10 seconds).

- Look, listen, and feel for breathing (a).
- If breathing, place victim in recovery position.
- If not breathing, give 2 slow rescue breaths (2 seconds each).
- If breaths do not cause the chest to rise, the airway may be blocked. Reposition the head and try breaths again. If chest does not rise, begin CPR (see step #6). When you open the airway to give a breath, look for an object in the throat and if seen, remove it.
- If two breaths cause the chest to rise, continue to step #5.

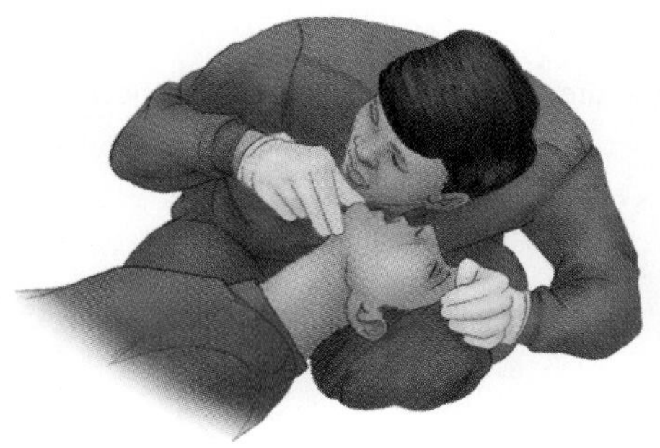

Check circulation (10 seconds).

Signs of circulation include—

- Breathing
- Coughing
- Movement

If not breathing, but other signs of circulation exist, give one breath every five seconds. Recheck signs of circulation every minute.

If no signs of circulation, begin CPR (step #6).

Basic Life Support
Adult and Child Rescue Breathing and CPR

6

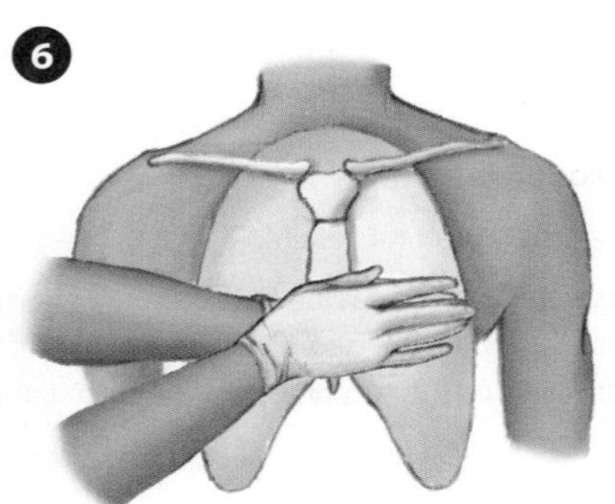

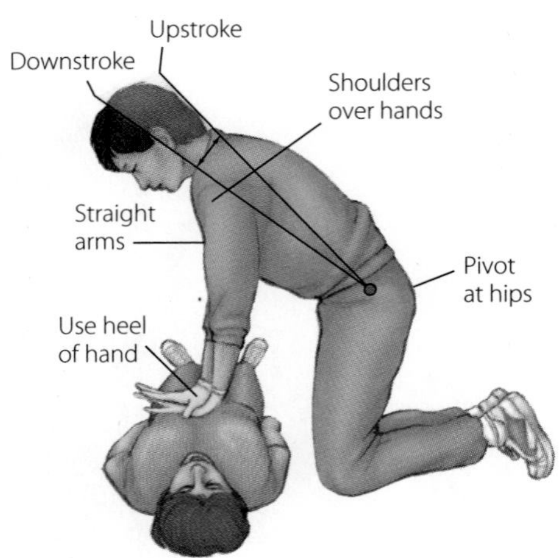

Perform CPR

- Place heel of one hand on the center of the chest between the nipples (lower half of the sternum).
- Using two hands, depress chest downward $1^1/_2$ to 2 inches.
- Give 15 chest compressions at a rate of about 100 per minute.
- Open the airway and give two slow breaths (two seconds each).
- Repeat cycles of 15 chest compressions and two rescue breaths until an AED is available (see AED information on page 19).

7

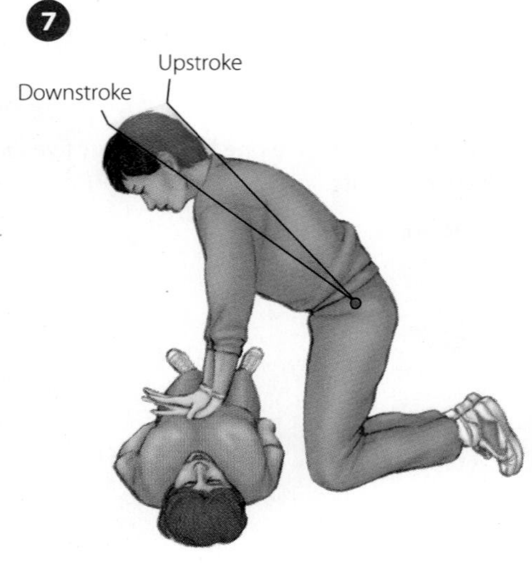

Recheck circulation

After four cycles of compressions and breaths (about one minute), recheck for signs of circulation.

- If not breathing and no other signs of circulation exist, resume CPR.

Basic Life Support
Adult and Child Rescue Breathing and CPR

7

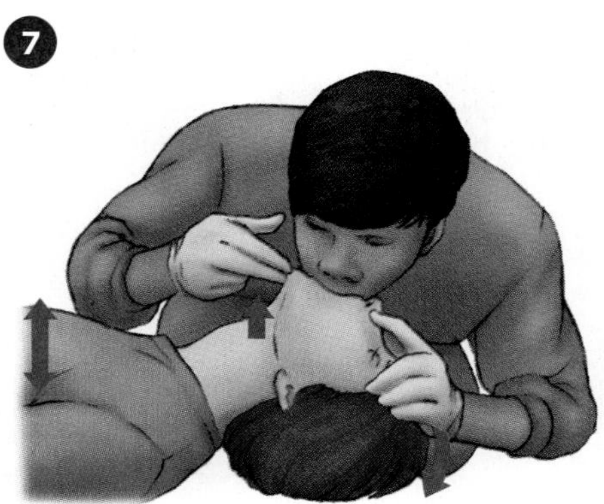

- If breathing, place victim in recovery position.
- **If not breathing, but other signs of circulation exist, provide one rescue breath about every five seconds.**
- Recheck for signs of circulation every few minutes.

8

Early defibrillation

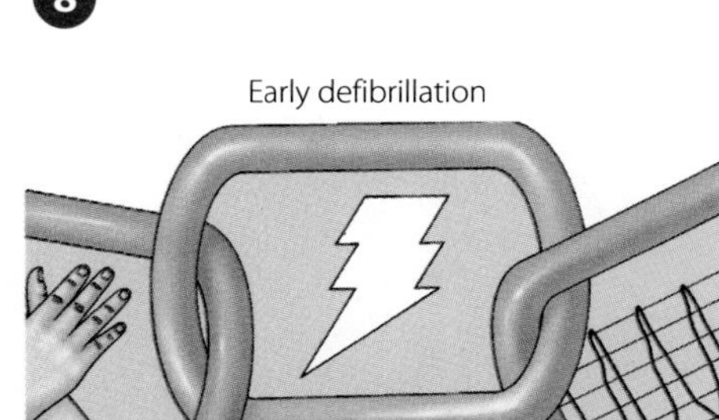

If you are trained to use an AED, follow this sequence:

- Perform CPR until an AED is available.
- Turn on the AED.
- Attach AED pads.
- "Analyze" the heart rhythm.
- Shock (up to three times if advised by AED).

After three shocks or after any AED prompt of "no shock indicated":

- Check for signs of circulation (including pulse).
- If no signs of circulation, perform CPR for one minute.

Check for signs of circulation. If absent:

- "Analyze" and follow the AED's prompts.
- Shock, if prompted.
- Repeat steps 6 and 7.
- Note – To use an AED on a child requires special electrode pads and reduced energy level.

Basic Life Support
Responsive Adult and Child Airway Obstruction

If person is responsive and cannot speak, breathe, or cough...

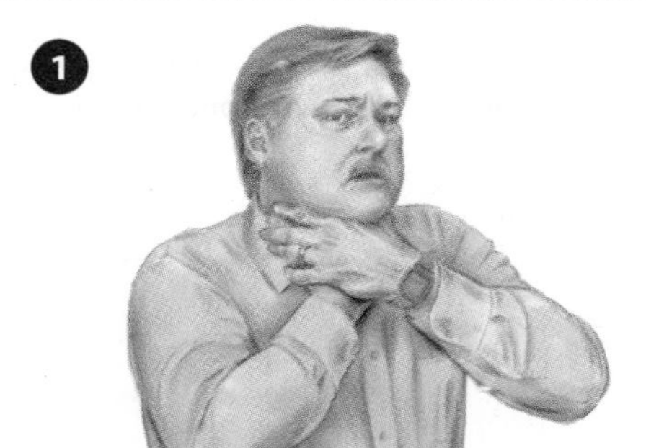

1. **Check victim for choking.**

- Ask "Are you choking? Can you speak?"
- A choking victim cannot speak, breathe, or cough and may clutch the neck with one or both hands.

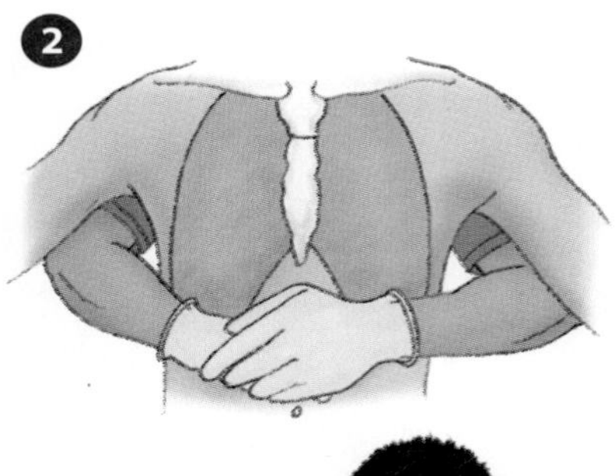

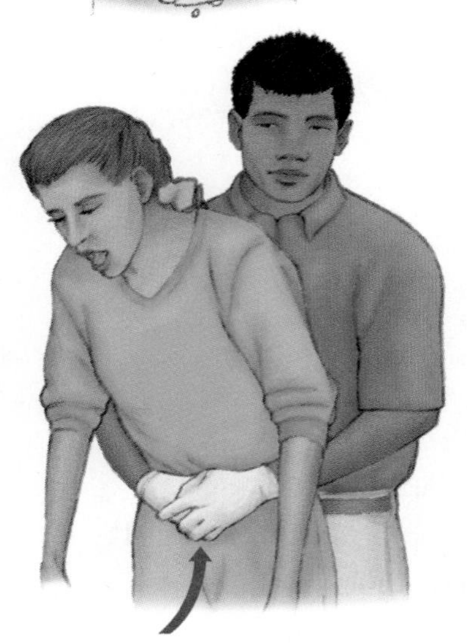

2. **Give abdominal thrusts** (Heimlich maneuver)

- Place a fist against the victim's abdomen just above the navel.
- Grasp the fist with your other hand and press into victim's abdomen with quick inward and upward thrusts.
- Continue thrusts until object is removed or victim becomes unresponsive.

Give chest thrusts instead of abdominal thrusts for women in late stages of pregnancy or large victims.

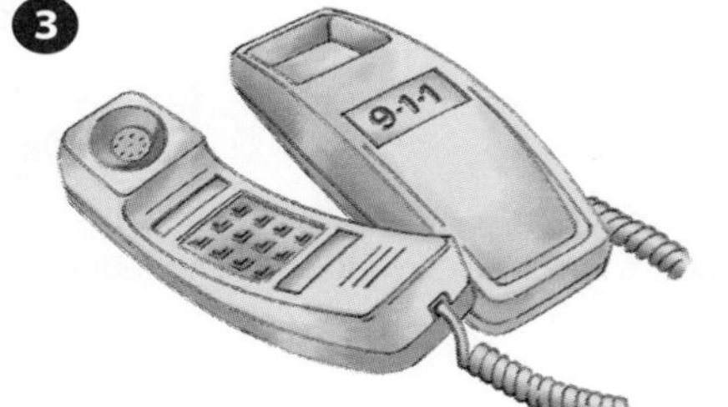

3. **If the victim becomes unresponsive**

- Call 9-1-1 or emergency telephone number to activate the EMS system (or send someone to do it).
- Assess the victim and begin CPR if needed.
- Each time you open the airway to give a breath, look for an object in the throat and if seen, remove it.

Differences Between Adult and Child (1 – 8 years) Basic Life Support

IF child ...	THEN ...
Is unresponsive and rescuer is alone	***activate the EMS system after one minute of resuscitation*** (in adults, activate EMS immediately after determining unresponsiveness).
Is ***not*** breathing but other signs of circulation exist	• give ***1 to 1 1/2 second breaths*** (in adults give 1 1/2 to 2 second breaths). • give ***one breath every 3 seconds*** (in adults give one breath every 5 seconds).
does ***not*** have any signs of circulation 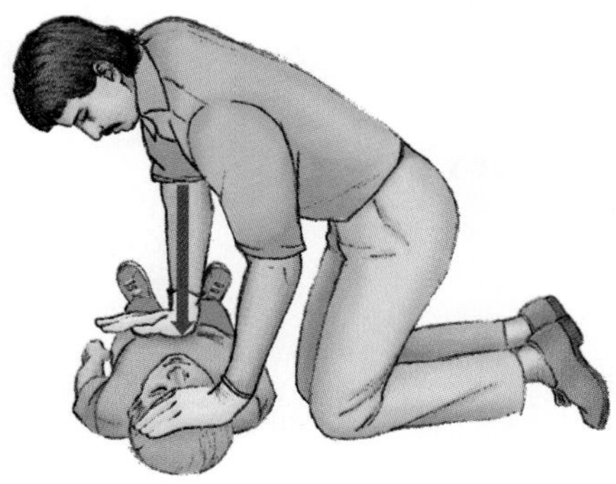	• give ***chest compressions with one hand*** (hand nearest feet) while keeping other hand on child's forehead (adult requires two hands on victim's chest for compressions). • give ***one breath after every 5 chest compressions*** (adult CPR requires two breaths after every 15 compressions). • Children up to 8 years of age and 55 pounds (25 kg) can be defibrillated with an AED. This requires special equipment and a reduced energy level.

Adult Basic Life Support Proficiency Checklist

S = self check / P = partner check / I = instructor check

Adult Rescue Breathing

	S	P	I
1. Check responsiveness.	○	○	○
2. Activate EMS.	○	○	○
3. Airway open.	○	○	○
4. Breathing check.	○	○	○
5. 2 slow breaths.	○	○	○
6. Check circulation.	○	○	○
7. Rescue breathing (1 every 5 seconds).	○	○	○
8. Recheck circulation and breathing after first minute, then every few minutes.	○	○	○

Adult CPR

	S	P	I
1. Check responsiveness.	○	○	○
2. Activate EMS.	○	○	○
3. Airway open.	○	○	○
4. Breathing check.	○	○	○
5. 2 slow breaths.	○	○	○
6. Check circulation.	○	○	○
7. Position hands.	○	○	○
8. 15 compressions.	○	○	○
9. 2 slow breaths.	○	○	○
10. Continue CPR (3 more cycles, for total of 4).	○	○	○
11. Recheck circulation.	○	○	○
12. Continue CPR.	○	○	○
13. Recheck circulation every few minutes.	○	○	○

Adult Choking

	S	P	I
1. Position hands.	○	○	○
2. Give abdominal thrusts until the object is removed or the victim is unresponsive.	○	○	○
3. If unresponsive, assess victim and begin CPR if needed.	○	○	○

Child Basic Life Support Proficiency Checklist

S = self check / P = partner check / I = instructor check

Child Rescue Breathing

	S	P	I
1. Check responsiveness.	O	O	O
2. Send a bystander, if available, to call EMS.	O	O	O
3. **A**irway open.	O	O	O
4. **B**reathing check.	O	O	O
5. 2 slow breaths.	O	O	O
6. **C**heck circulation.	O	O	O
7. Rescue breathing (1 every 3 seconds).	O	O	O
8. If alone, call EMS after 1 minute.	O	O	O
9. Recheck circulation and breathing after first minute, then every few minutes.	O	O	O

Child CPR

	S	P	I
1. Check responsiveness.	O	O	O
2. Send a bystander, if available, to call EMS.	O	O	O
3. Airway open.	O	O	O
4. Breathing check.	O	O	O
5. 2 slow breaths.	O	O	O
6. Check circulation.	O	O	O
7. Position hand.	O	O	O
8. 5 compressions with 1 hand.	O	O	O
9. 1 slow breath.	O	O	O
10. Continue CPR for 1 minute (19 more cycles, for total of 20).	O	O	O
11. If alone, call EMS after 1 minute.	O	O	O
12. Recheck circulation.	O	O	O
13. Continue CPR.	O	O	O
14. Recheck circulation every few minutes.	O	O	O

Child Choking

	S	P	I
1. Postion hands.	O	O	O
2. Give abdominal thrusts until the object is removed or the victim is unresponsive.	O	O	O
3. If unresponsive, assess victim and begin CPR if needed.	O	O	O

Learning Activities

Adult and Child Basic Life Support

Directions: Circle Yes if you agree with the statement, and circle No if you disagree.

Yes No **1.** You should give one rescue breath every 3 seconds when performing rescue breathing for an adult.

Yes No **2.** Adult CPR requires 15 compressions and 2 breaths, while child CPR requires 5 compressions and 1 breath.

Yes No **3.** An unresponsive, breathing victim should be placed in the recovery position.

Yes No **4.** When performing rescue breathing, breathe forcefully to make sure the chest rises quickly.

Yes No **5.** If a person can cough forcefully, he or she is choking and needs the Heimlich maneuver.

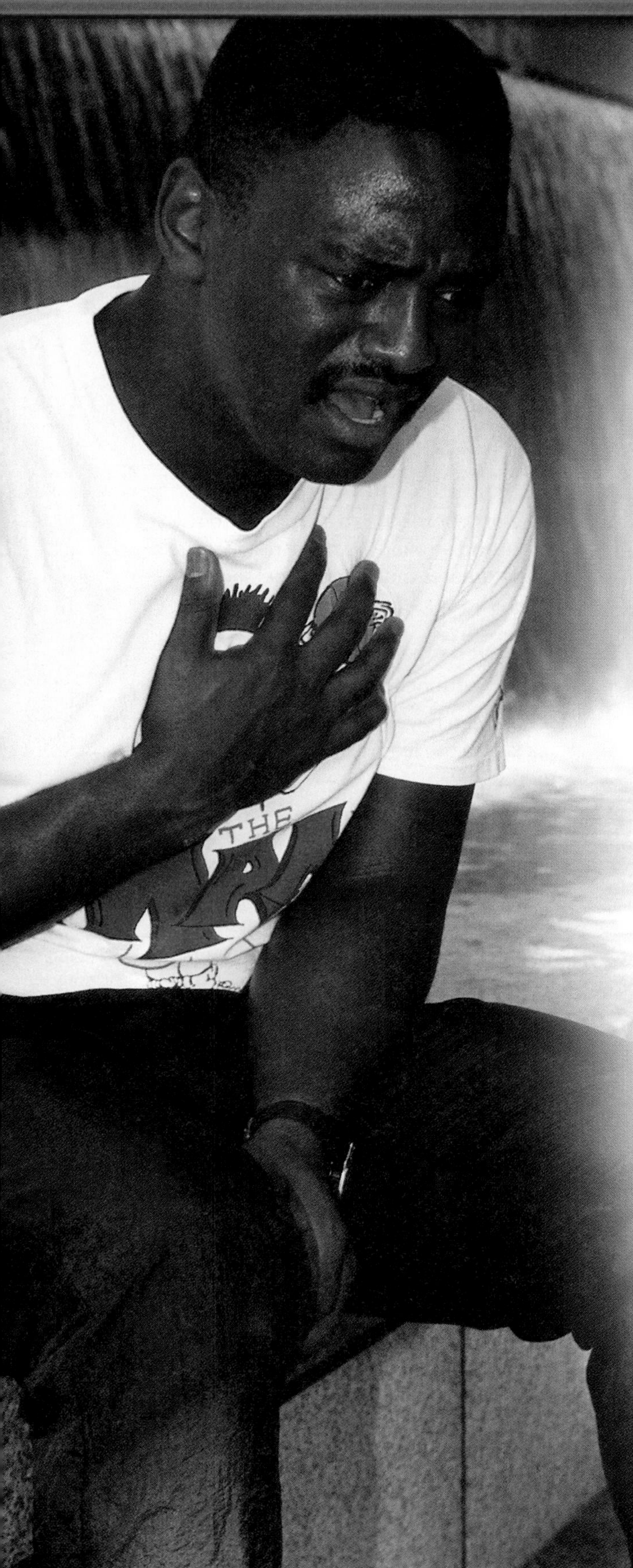

Chapter 4

Cardiovascular Emergencies

Heart Attack

A heart attack occurs when the blood supply to part of the heart muscle is severely reduced or stopped. This often occurs when the coronary arteries (the arteries that supply blood to the heart muscle) are blocked by an obstruction or a spasm.

What to Look For

Heart attacks are difficult to determine. Because medical care at the onset of a heart attack is vital to survival and the quality of recovery, if you suspect a heart attack for any reason, seek medical attention *at once.*

The possible signs and symptoms of a heart attack include:

- uncomfortable pressure, fullness, squeezing, or pain in the center of the chest that lasts more than a few minutes or that goes away and comes back (►Table 1).
- pain spreading to the arms, shoulders, neck, jaw, or back.
- chest discomfort with lightheadedness, fainting, sweating, nausea, shortness of breath, or rapid, irregular heartbeat.

Not all these warning signs and symptoms occur in every heart attack. Many victims will deny that they might be experiencing something as serious as a heart attack. Don't take "no" for an answer. Delay can seriously increase the risk of major damage. Insist on taking prompt action.

Victims who are brought to a hospital by ambulance receive clot-dissolving drugs (thombolytics) sooner than those arriving by other means. It is clear that reducing the time from the onset of a heart attack to the receiving of thrombolytic drugs is beneficial and decreases the amount of heart damage.

What to Do

1. Call 9-1-1 to get to the nearest hospital emergency department that offers 24-hour emergency cardiovascular care.

2. Monitor the ABCs. Give CPR if necessary.
3. Help the victim to the most comfortable position, usually sitting with legs up and bent at the knees. Loosen any restrictive clothing. Be calm and reassuring.
4. Assist with any prescribed medication such as nitroglycerin. Aspirin has also been shown to be helpful.

Cardiac Arrest

Cardiac arrest is the sudden, unexpected stoppage of the pumping action of the heart leading to inadequate circulation to maintain life. Signs include sudden unresponsiveness, and absent breathing.

No breathing for several minutes can lead to cardiac arrest. Drowning, suffocation, airway obstruction, certain drugs, and asthma are reasons breathing may stop.

Cardiac arrest can occur because of a heart attack, electrocution, drowning, or electrolyte imbalance.

Victims have the best chance of surviving if (►Table 2):

- CPR is started promptly and
- They receive early defibrillation within three to five minutes.

Brain damage begins after four to six minutes and is certain after 10 minutes when no CPR is given.

CPR is not effective if livor mortis or rigor mortis is present. Livor mortis is the dull red discoloration of the skin resulting from accumulation of blood in the veins about 20 to 30 minutes after death. Rigor mortis is the

Table 1: Chest Pain

Cause of Pain	Characteristics	Care
Muscle or rib pain from exercise or injury	Reproduced by movement Tender spot when pressed	Rest Aspirin or ibuprofen
Respiratory infection (pneumonia, bronchitis, pleuritis)	Cough Fever Sore throat Production of sputum	Antibiotics
Indigestion	Belching Heartburn Nausea Sour taste	Antacids
Angina	Lasts <10 minutes	Rest Victim's nitroglycerin
Heart attack (myocardial infarction)	Lasts >10 minutes Pressure, squeezing, or pain in center of chest Pain spreads to shoulders, neck, or arms, jaw, back Lightheadedness, fainting, sweating, nausea, shortness of breath	Call EMS Check ABCs Rest Victim's nitroglycerin

Risk Factors of Cardiovascular Disease

Several factors contribute to an increased risk of heart attack and stroke. The more risk factors present, the greater the chance a person will develop heart disease.

Risk factors you cannot change:

- Heredity. Tendencies appear in family lines.
- Male sex. Men have a greater risk, although heart attack is also the leading cause of death among women.
- Age. Most heart attack victims are 65 or older.

Risk factors you can change or control:

- Cigarette smoking. Smokers have more than twice the risk of heart attack as nonsmokers.
- High blood pressure. This condition adds to the heart's workload.
- High blood cholesterol level. Too much cholesterol in the blood can cause a buildup on the walls of the arteries.
- Diabetes. This condition affects the blood's cholesterol and triglyceride levels.
- Obesity. Being overweight influences blood pressure and blood cholesterol, can result in diabetes, and can put an added strain on the heart.
- Physical inactivity. Inactive people have twice the risk of heart attack as active people.
- Stress. All people feel stress but react in different ways. Excessive, long-term stress may create problems in some people.

Table 2: Chances of Survival (Survival Rate %)

	Time Until Advanced Cardiac Life Support Begins		
	<8 min.	**8-16 min.**	**>16 min.**
Time Until Basic Life Support (CPR)			
< 4 min.	43%	19%	10%
4–8 min.	27%	19%	6%
> 8 min.	N/A	7%	0%

Source: National Ski Patrol, based upon Eisenberg, et al., *JAMA*, 1979, 241:1905–1907.

stiffening of the muscles and is caused by chemical changes in the muscles. It appears from 30 minutes to six hours or more after death, most commonly within two to four hours. Do not confuse it with severe hypothermia. Severe injuries and other conditions incompatible with life are also reasons for not starting CPR. Previously agreed upon do-not-resuscitate (DNR) or no-CPR orders can become a factor in not starting CPR, especially in hospitals and nursing homes.

Stroke

A stroke occurs when there is a disruption of blood supply to the brain, such as when the cerebral arteries that supply the brain with blood are blocked or rupture.

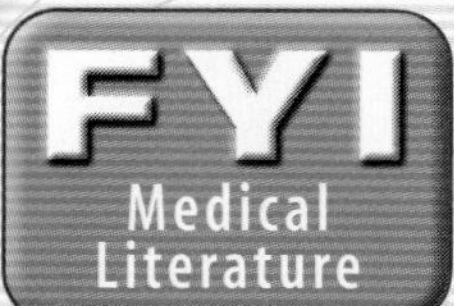

Strenuous Exertion: Not for the Sedentary

Researchers interviewed 1,228 people hospitalized after a heart attack. Only 5 percent said their heart attack symptoms started within an hour of heavy exertion (lifting, pushing, jogging, gardening, chopping wood), but most of those who had heart attacks during physical exertion exercised less than once a week. People who exercised several times a week had double the risk of heart attack during the hours after heavy exertion, as compared with periods of light exertion. But for sedentary individuals, the risk of heart attack was 107 times higher during strenuous exertion. Thus, frequent exercise lowers the risk of heart attack and lowers the risk that strenuous exertion will trigger a heart attack.

Source: M. A. Mittlemen et al., "Triggering of Acute Myocardial Infarction by Heavy Exertion," *New England Journal of Medicine* 329(23):1677 (Dec. 1993).

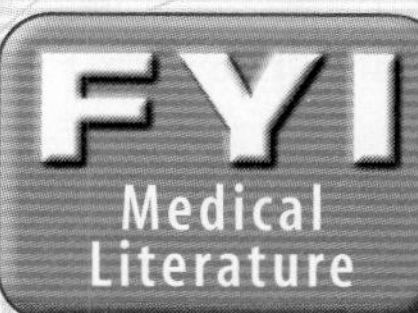

Monday Morning Heart Attacks

Studies show that heart attacks occur most frequently in the morning and during the winter months. In one study, 5,596 heart attacks and sudden cardiac deaths were recorded in Augsburg, Germany, from 1958 through 1990. The increased heart attack risk was highest among people employed outside the home, especially in blue collar jobs, when heart attack incidence peaked on Mondays. Sundays had the lowest heart attack rate for all workers. There was no significant daily variation in heart attacks among non-working people.

Source: S. N. Willich et al., "Weekly Variation of Acute Myocardial Infarction," *Circulation* 90:87 (July 1994).

What to Look for

The signs and symptoms of stroke include:

- Sudden onset of severe headache
- Loss of responsiveness
- Blurred or decreased vision, especially in one eye
- Problems speaking or understanding
- Weakness, numbness, or paralysis of the face (facial droop), an arm, or a leg on one side of the body.

What to Do

To care for a stroke:

- Call 9-1-1
- Loosen any restrictive clothing
- Place the victim in the recovery position
- If unresponsive, check the ABCs.

Learning Activities

Cardiovascular Emergencies

Directions: Circle Yes if you agree with the statement, and circle No if you disagree.

Yes No **1.** Persistent chest pain/pressure is a primary signal of a heart attack.

Yes No **2.** To care for a possible heart attack victim, allow him or her to rest in the most comfortable position.

Yes No **3.** The signs of stroke include facial droop and abnormal speech.

Yes No **4.** A stroke victim should be placed flat on his or her back until EMS personnel arrive.

Yes No **5.** Heredity is a cardiovascular disease risk factor that can be changed.

Chapter 5

Infant Basic Life Support

Basic life support techniques for an infant (under one year) differ only slightly from those for an adult or child. Initially occurring cardiac arrest in infants is rare. Like children, infants also have a respiratory arrest with cardiac arrest developing later because the heart muscle did not receive sufficient oxygen.

Infant Rescue Breathing and CPR

Responsiveness

The first priority in cardiopulmonary emergency is to determine the infant's responsiveness. This is done by tapping the infant and speaking loudly. If basic life support is necessary, give resuscitation for one minute before activating the EMS. The rescuer should shout for help if alone.

Properly position the infant so that if any resuscitation efforts are needed, they can be performed. If the infant is found lying facedown, turn the infant as a complete unit onto his or her back. The infant's head and neck should always be supported with one of your hands so that they remain aligned with the rest of the body and do not twist.

A: Airway

After unresponsiveness has been determined and the infant has been properly positioned, open the airway by using the head-tilt/chin-lift method. To do this, place one hand to apply pressure on the infant's forehead to gently tilt the head backward. Do not overtilt the head backward because it can block the airway because of the pliability of the infant's tissues. To lift the chin, place the finger(s) of your other hand under the bony part of the jaw. Then lift your fingers to bring the chin up. The fingers should not press on the soft tissue under the infant's chin because it can interfere with the opening of the airway. While the chin is lifted, the hand on the forehead maintains the head-tilt position of the infant. Sometimes, opening the airway may be all that is necessary for the infant to breathe.

When a spinal injury is suspected, open the airway using the jaw thrust without tilting the head back. If the airway remains blocked, tilt the head slowly and gently until the airway is open. This technique for a suspected spinal-injured infant will help minimize any existing injury. While stabilizing the head, place the fingers of each hand behind the angles of the infant's lower jaw on each side of the head and move the lower jaw forward without tilting the head backward; however, it may be necessary to tilt the head slightly if the airway cannot be opened.

B: Breathing

After unresponsiveness has been determined and the airway has been opened, you should look, listen, and feel for breathing. You should (1) look to see whether there is any visible movement of the infant's chest, (2) listen for air by placing your ear next to the infant's mouth and nose, and (3) feel for air by placing your cheek next to the infant's mouth and nose. If breathing is present, you will see the infant's chest rise and fall, hear air coming from the infant's mouth and nose, and feel air against your own cheek.

Rescue Breathing

The breaths for an infant should be limited to the amount needed to raise the chest. For infants, use shallow puffs of air.

To perform rescue breathing for an infant, follow these steps:

1. Open the airway.
2. Form an airtight seal over the infant's nose and mouth (or nose only).
3. Give two breaths using shallow puffs of air.
4. Watch to see if the infant's chest rises.
5. Remove your mouth to allow the air to come out and move your head away as you take another breath.

If breaths do not go in after repositioning the head, begin CPR as indicated in the skill sheets beginning on page 34.

If the infant is not breathing, but has other signs of circulation, continue rescue breathing. Because infants breathe faster than adults, breathe into an infant once every three seconds or 20 times a minute. Between breaths, remove your mouth from the infant's to allow air to flow out of the infant's lungs. As you remove your mouth, you should turn your head to the side to see if the infant's chest fell after each breath. For rescue breathing, breathe into the infant slowly, just enough to make the chest gently rise.

Gastric Distention

Rescue breaths tend to cause stomach or gastric distention more often in infants than in adults. Minimize this problem by limiting the breaths to the amount needed to make the chest rise. Avoid overinflating the lungs. Gastric distention can cause regurgitation and aspiration of stomach contents.

C: Circulation

After a nonbreathing infant has been given two breaths, check for signs of circulation.

If signs of circulation exist, but breathing is absent, continue rescue breathing. A rescue breath is given once every three seconds or 20 times a minute. After 20 breaths, you should activate EMS.

If there are no signs of circulation, begin CPR until a defibrillator is available. The proper chest compression point in an infant is the midsternum. To locate this area, imagine a line connecting the infant's nipples. Place three fingers (index, middle, and ring) with the index finger next to the imaginary nipple line on the infant's feet side. Lift the index finger off the chest (▼Figure 1).

Use the two remaining fingers to apply the chest compressions. Press the infant's midsternum (area between the nipples) 1/2 to 1 inch into the chest with the middle and ring finger. Either place your other hand under the infant's shoulder to provide support or keep it on the infant's forehead to keep the head tilted. If the infant is carried during CPR, the length of the body is on the rescuer's forearm with the head kept level with the trunk.

An infant's heart rate is faster than an adult's and so the rate of compressions must also be faster. The infant compression rate is at least 100 per minute. External chest compressions must always be combined with rescue breathing.

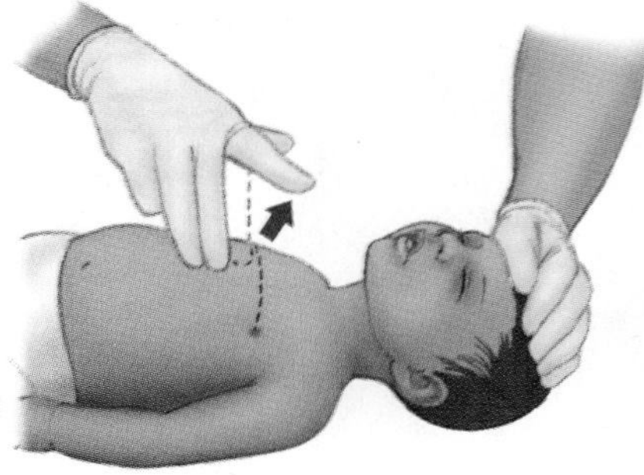

Figure 1 Proper finger placement for chest compressions.

Common Problems in Children and Infants

Airway Obstruction

- Partial airway obstruction (child or infant is alert and sitting):
  - High-pitched inhalation sound, crowing, or noisy breathing
  - Child is responsive
  - First aid: Allow position of comfort; assist young child to sit up (may sit on parent's lap); do not lay child or infant down
- Complete airway obstruction and altered mental status or cyanosis (blue skin color) and partial obstruction:
  - No crying or speaking and cyanosis
    a. Child's cough becomes ineffective
    b. Increased breathing difficulty accompanied by high-pitched inhalation sound
    c. Child or infant becomes unresponsive
    d. Altered mental status
  - First aid: Clear airway using either child foreign body obstruction procedures or infant foreign body obstruction procedures
- Attempt rescue breathing

Breathing Emergencies

- Breathing distress precedes respiratory failure and is indicated by any of the following:
  - Breathing rate >60 in infants
  - Breathing rate >30–40 in children
  - Nasal flaring
  - High-pitched inhalation sound
  - Cyanosis (blue skin color)
  - Altered mental status (eg, combative, unresponsive)
- Respiratory failure/arrest:
  - Breathing rate <10 per minute in child
  - Breathing rate <20 per minute in infant
  - Unresponsive
  - No pulse

Sudden Infant Death Syndrome (SIDS)

- Signs and symptoms:
  - Sudden death in the first year of life
  - Causes are not clearly understood
  - Baby is most commonly discovered in the early morning
- First aid:
  - Complete ABC assessment
  - Comfort, calm, and reassure the parents while awaiting EMS
    a. Try to resuscitate unless the baby is stiff
    b. Parents will be in agony from emotional distress, remorse, and guilt; avoid any comments that might suggest blame

Child Abuse

- Physical abuse and neglect are the two forms of child abuse:
  - Abuse: improper or excessive action so as to injure or cause harm
  - Neglect: giving insufficient attention or respect to someone who has a claim to that attention
- Signs and symptoms of abuse:
  - Multiple bruises in various stages of healing
  - Patterns of injury (eg, cigarette burns, whip mark, handprints)
  - Fresh burns such as scalding, untreated burns, body part dipped
  - Parents seen inappropriately unconcerned
  - Conflicting explanations of injury
- Signs and symptoms of neglect:
  - Lack of adult supervision
  - Malnourished-appearing child
  - Unsafe living environment
  - Untreated soft tissue injuries
- Do not accuse parents or guardians
- State law requires reporting:
  - Report what you see and what you hear
  - Do not comment on what you think

The ratio of compressions to breaths is 5 to 1. See the detailed skill sheets for CPR on pages 34–36 ►Skill Scan.

Airway Obstruction (Choking)

As discussed before, the airway may be partially or completely blocked. With a partial airway obstruction, an infant is able to make persistent coughing efforts that should not be hampered. If good air exchange becomes a poor exchange or poor air exchange occurs initially, the infant should be managed as having a complete airway obstruction. Poor air exchanges are indicated by ineffective coughing, high-pitched noises, breathing difficulty, and blueness of the lips and fingernail beds.

Choking management of a completely obstructed airway consists of the combination of back blows and chest thrusts. Abdominal thrusts are not advisable for infants because of possible injury to the abdominal organs. Any visible object can be removed from the mouth using a finger sweep.

Back Blows and Chest Thrusts

To perform back blows on an infants, straddle the infant facedown over your forearm. The infant's head should be lower than the trunk. Your hand should be around the jaw and neck of the infant giving support to the infant's head. For more support, rest your forearm under the infant on your thigh. Using the heel of the other hand, you

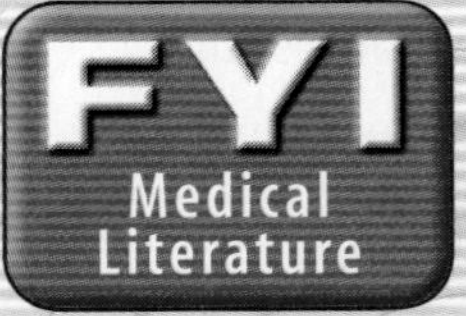

Facts About Sudden Infant Death Syndrome (SIDS)

Many more children die of SIDS in a year than all who die of cancer, heart disease, pneumonia, child abuse, AIDS, cystic fibrosis, and muscular dystrophy combined . . .

What Is SIDS?

- Sudden Infant Death Syndrome (SIDS) is a medical term that describes the sudden death of an infant that remains unexplained after all known and possible causes have been carefully ruled out through autopsy, death scene investigation, and review of the medical history. SIDS is responsible for more deaths than any other cause in childhood for babies one month to one year of age, claiming 150,000 victims in the United States in this generation alone—7,000 babies each year—*nearly one baby every hour of every day.* It strikes families of all races, ethnic, and socioeconomic origins without warning; neither parent nor physician can predict that something is going wrong. In fact, most SIDS victims appear healthy prior to death.

What Causes SIDS?

- While there are still no adequate medical explanations for SIDS deaths, current theories include: (1) stress in a normal baby, caused by infection or other factors; (2) a birth defect; (3) failure to develop; and/or (4) a critical period when all babies are especially vulnerable, such as a time of rapid growth.
- Many new studies have been launched to learn how and why SIDS occurs. Scientists are exploring the development and function of the nervous system, the brain, the heart, breathing and sleep patterns, body chemical balances, autopsy findings, and environmental factors. It is likely that SIDS, like many other medical disorders, will eventually have more than one explanation.

Can SIDS Be Prevented?

- No, not yet. But, some recent studies have begun to isolate several risk factors that, though not causes of SIDS in and of themselves, may play a role in some cases. (*It is important that, since the causes of SIDS remain unknown, SIDS parents refrain from concluding that their child care practices may have caused their baby's death.*)

Some Basic Facts about SIDS:

- SIDS is a definite medical entity and is the major cause of death in infants after the first month of life.
- SIDS claims the lives of over 7,000 American babies each year . . . *nearly one baby every hour of every day.*
- SIDS victims appear to be healthy prior to death.
- Currently, SIDS cannot be predicted or prevented, even by a physician.
- There appears to be no suffering; death occurs very rapidly, usually during sleep.

What SIDS Is Not:

- SIDS is **not** caused by external suffocation.
- SIDS is **not** caused by vomiting and choking.
- SIDS is **not** contagious.
- SIDS does **not** cause pain or suffering in the infant.
- SIDS can**not** be predicted.

Source: SIDS Network. Used with permission.

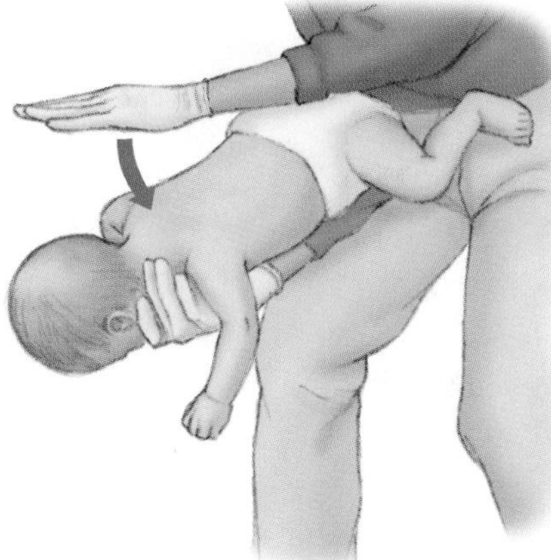

Figure 2 Give 5 back blows.

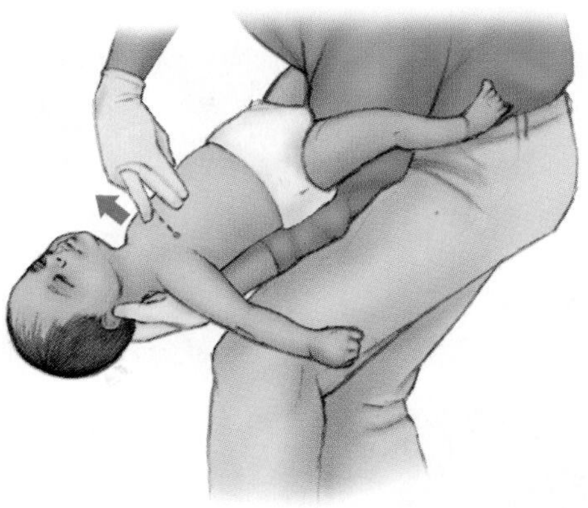

Figure 3 Give 5 chest thrusts.

are ready to give five rapid back blows between the infant's shoulder blades (▲**Figure 2**).

To give chest thrusts, turn the infant onto his or her back. After delivering the five back blows, immediately place your free hand on the back of the infant's head and neck while the other hand remains in place. Using both hands and forearms to sandwich the infant—one supporting the jaw, neck, and chest, and the other the back—turn the infant over. Once turned onto the back, the infant should be resting on your thigh. The infant's head should be lower than the trunk. With the infant positioned, give five chest thrusts in rapid succession. The thrusts are given to the sternum (between the nipples), using two fingers. The technique used to locate and perform thrusts is the same as that used to perform external chest compressions for CPR (▲**Figure 3**). See the skill sheet for Infant Airway Obstruction on page 37.

If the choking infant becomes unresponsive, shout for help and begin CPR. Look for the object. If seen, remove it. If the infant is not breathing, give one breath, retilt head and give a second breath. If there are no signs of circulation, after the first two breaths, begin chest compressions. The sequence of actions: open airway, look for an object (if seen remove it), give one breath, 5 chest compressions. Repeat sequence for about one minute and if you are alone, phone 911.

Basic Life Support
Infant Rescue Breathing and CPR

If you see a motionless infant ...

1

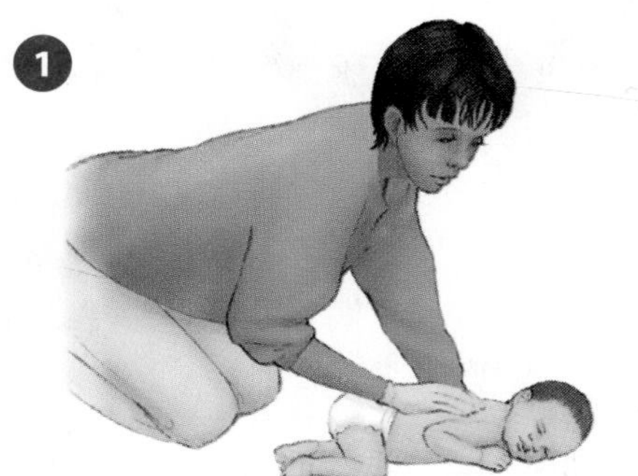

Check responsiveness

- Tap the victim and shout, "Are you okay?"

2

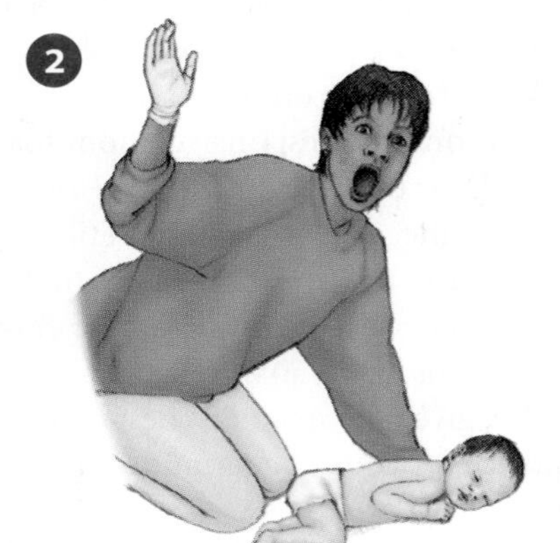

Activate EMS

- Ask a bystander to call the local emergency telephone number, usually 9-1-1.
- If you are alone, call EMS after one minute of resuscitation, unless a bystander can be sent.

3

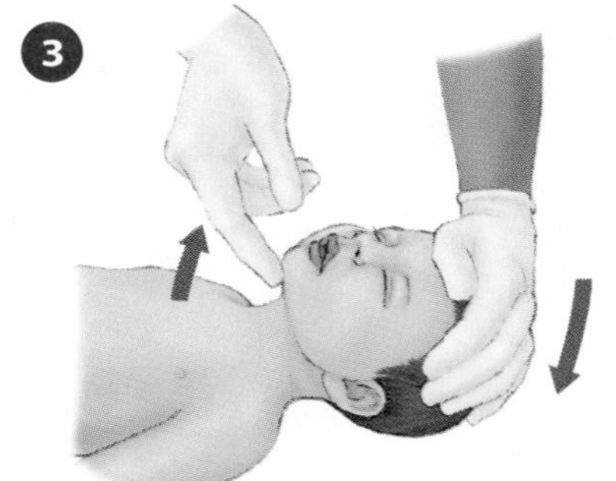

Open the airway (use head-tilt/chin-lift method)

- Place your hand that is nearest victim's head on victim's forehead and tilt head back slightly.
- Place the fingers of your other hand under the chin and lift gently. Avoid pressing on the soft tissues under the jaw.

4

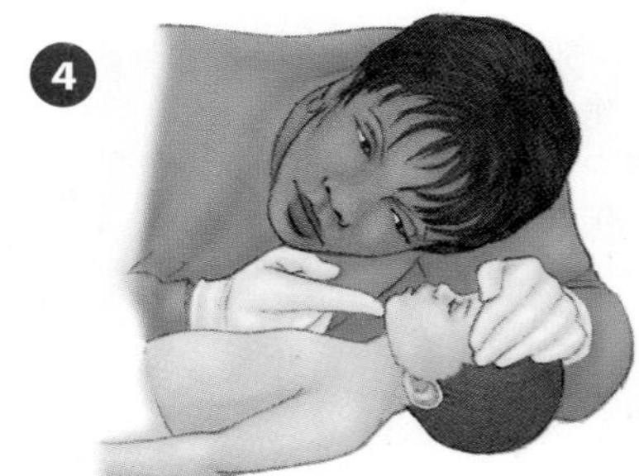

Check for breathing (10 seconds)

- Place your ear over the victim's mouth and nose while keeping the airway open.
- *Look* at the victim's chest to check for rise and fall; *listen* and *feel* for breathing.

Basic Life Support
Infant Rescue Breathing and CPR

5

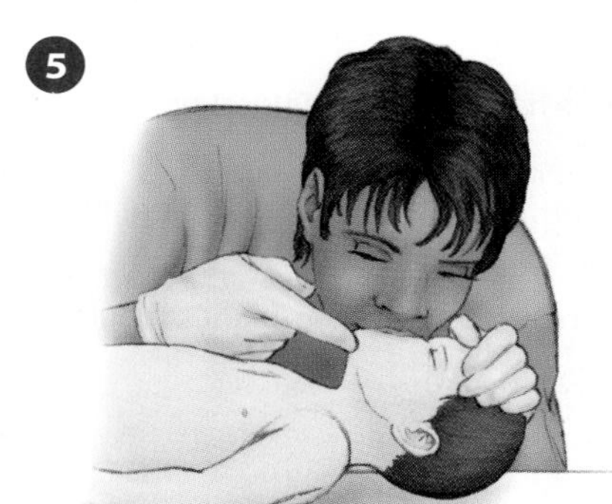

If not breathing, give 2 slow breaths

- Keep the airway open.
- Take a breath and place your mouth over the victim's mouth and nose, or nose only.
- Each breath 1–1 1/2 seconds.
- Watch chest rise to see if your breaths go in.
- Allow for chest deflation after each breath.

If breaths do not go in

Retilt the head and try again.

If unsuccessful give CPR. Each time you open the airway, look for an object in the throat, and if seen, remove it.

6

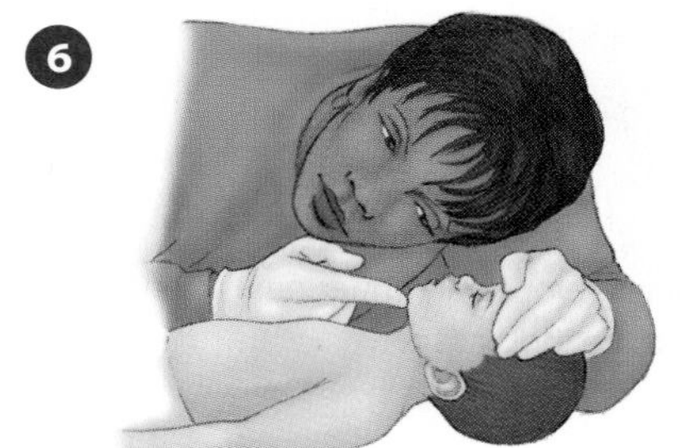

Check for signs of circulation (10 seconds)

Signs of circulation include:

- Breathing
- Coughing
- Movement

7

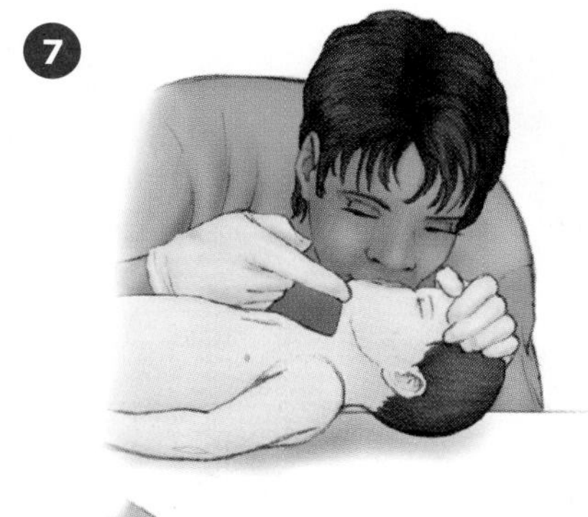

If no breathing, but other signs of circulation

- Give 1 breath every 3 seconds.
- Recheck signs of circulation every minute.

If there are no signs of circulation

- Begin CPR.
    1. Place 2-3 fingers in the center of the chest.
    2. Compress the chest 5 times.
    3. Push sternum straight down $\frac{1}{2}$ to 1 inch.
    4. Compress the chest at a rate of at least 100 compressions per minute.
- Give 1 slow breath.
- Continue cycles of 5 compressions and 1 breath for 1 minute, then check for signs of circulation. If absent, restart CPR with chest compressions. Recheck the signs of circulation every few minutes. If there are signs of circulation but no breathing, give rescue breathing.
- Note – To use an AED on an infant requires special electrode pads and reduced energy level.

Basic Life Support
Infant Airway Obstruction

If infant is responsive and cannot cry, breathe or cough...

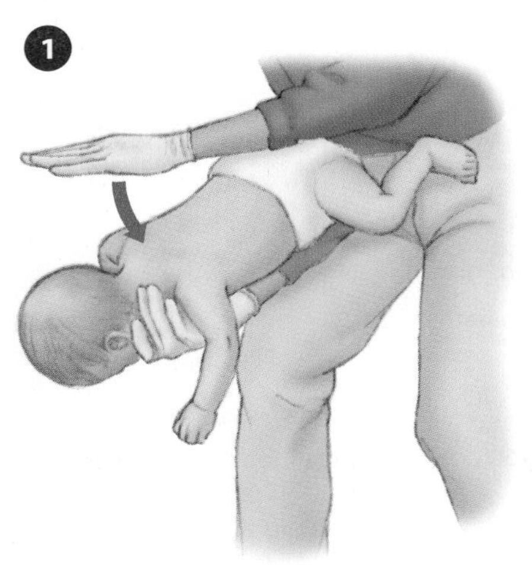

1 Give up to 5 back blows

- Hold the infant's head and neck with one hand by firmly supporting the infant's jaw between your thumb and fingers.
- Lay the infant facedown over your forearm with head lower than his or her chest. Brace your forearm and the infant against your thigh.
- Give up to 5 distinct and separate back blows between the infant's shoulder blades with the heel of your hand.

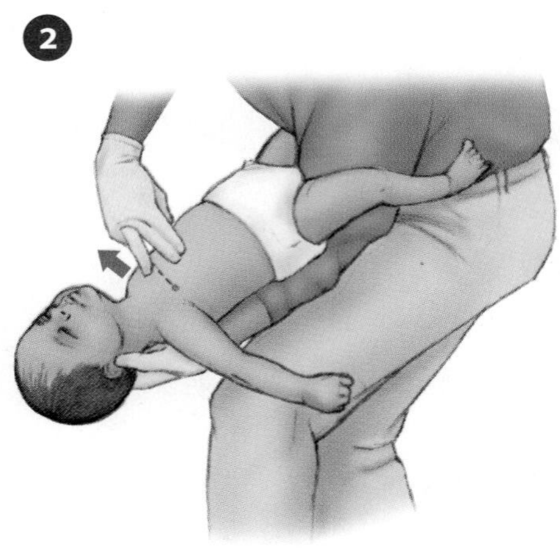

2 Give up to 5 chest thrusts

- While supporting the back of the infant's head, roll the infant face up.
- Place 3 fingers on the infant's sternum with your ring finger next to and below the imaginary nipple line toward the infant's feet.
- Lift your ring finger off the chest.
- Give up to 5 separate and distinct thrusts with your index and middle fingers on the infant's sternum in a manner similar to CPR chest compressions, but at a slower rate.

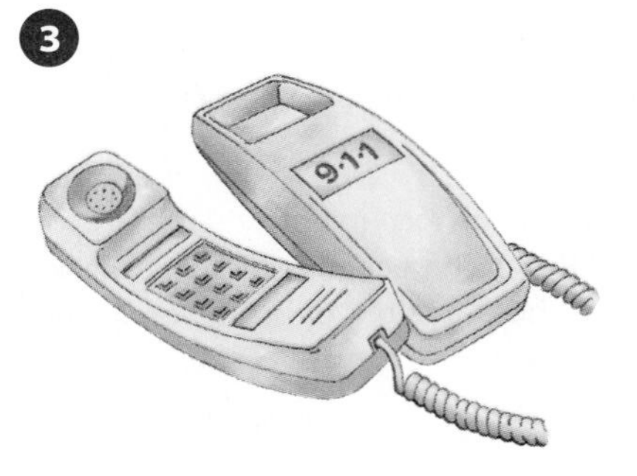

3 Repeat

- Until the infant becomes unresponsive. Call 9-1-1, assess the infant, and begin CPR if needed. Each time you open the airway to give a breath, look for an object in the throat and if seen, remove it.

OR

- Until the object is expelled, and infant begins to breathe or cough forcefully.

Infant Basic Life Support Proficiency Checklist

S = self check / P = partner check / I = instructor check

Infant Rescue Breathing

	S	P	I
1. Check responsiveness.	O	O	O
2. Send a bystander, if available, to call EMS.	O	O	O
3. **A**irway open.	O	O	O
4. **B**reathing check.	O	O	O
5. 2 slow breaths.	O	O	O
6. **C**heck circulation.	O	O	O
7. Rescue breathing (1 every 3 seconds).	O	O	O
8. If alone, call EMS after 1 minute.	O	O	O
9. Recheck circulation and breathing after first minute, then every few minutes.	O	O	O

Infant CPR

	S	P	I
1. Check responsiveness.	O	O	O
2. Send a bystander, if available, to call EMS.	O	O	O
3. Airway open.	O	O	O
4. Breathing check.	O	O	O
5. 2 slow breaths.	O	O	O
6. Check circulation.	O	O	O
7. Position fingers.	O	O	O
8. 5 compressions with 2–3 fingers.	O	O	O
9. 1 slow breath.	O	O	O
10. Continue CPR for 1 minute.	O	O	O
11. If alone, call EMS after 1 minute.	O	O	O
12. Recheck circulation.	O	O	O
13. Continue CPR.	O	O	O
14. Recheck circulation every few minutes.	O	O	O

Infant Choking

	S	P	I
1. 5 back blows	O	O	O
2. 5 chest thrusts until the object is removed or the victim is unresponsive.	O	O	O
3. If unresponsive, assess victim, give CPR if needed.	O	O	O

Learning Activities

Infant Basic Life Support

Directions: Circle Yes if you agree with the statement, and circle No if you disagree.

Yes No **1.** To open an infant's airway, tilt the head back further than you would for an adult.

Yes No **2.** Abdominal thrusts are used to clear an airway obstruction in an infant.

Yes No **3.** Breathing emergencies are more common than cardiovascular emergencies in infants.

Yes No **4.** During infant CPR, compress the chest 1/2 to 1 inch, at a rate of at least 100 times per minute.

Yes No **5.** If you are alone, provide one minute of care for a nonbreathing infant before calling EMS.

Appendix A Basic Life Support Review

These techniques are the same for all victims regardless of age:

- Check responsiveness—tap and shout.
- Open airway—head-tilt/chin-lift; for suspected spinal injury use jaw-thrust without head-tilt.
- Check breathing—look at chest to rise and fall and listen and feel for breathing.
- If breathing, place in recovery position.
- If not breathing, give 2 slow breaths (#1 in table).
- If breaths did not cause chest to rise, retilt head and give breaths again.
- If breaths still unsuccessful, give CPR (#2 in table).
- Check for signs of circulation (breathing, coughing, movement, normal skin condition).
- If not breathing but other signs of circulation exist, give rescue breaths (#3 in table).
- If not breathing and if no other signs of circulation exist, give CPR (#4 in table).

Action	Adult (>8 years)	Child (1-8 years)	Infant (<1 year)
1. Breathing methods	Mouth-to-barrier device Mouth-to-mouth Mouth-to-nose Mouth-to-stoma	Mouth-to-barrier device Mouth-to-mouth Mouth-to-nose	Mouth-to-barrier device Mouth-to-mouth and nose Mouth-to-nose
2. Foreign-body airway obstruction in unresponsive victim	CPR cycles of 15 compressions to 2 breaths. Before giving a breath, look for an object in throat and if seen, remove it.	CPR cycles of 5 compressions to 1 breath. Before giving a breath, look for an object in throat and if seen, remove it.	CPR cycles of 5 compressions to 1 breath. Before giving a breath, look for an object in throat and if seen, remove it.
3. Rescue breathing	1 breath every 5 seconds. Should cause chest to rise.	1 breath every 3 seconds. Should cause chest to rise.	1 breath every 3 seconds. Should cause chest to rise.
4. Compressions:			
• Locating hand positions	• Center of chest, between nipples	• Center of chest, between nipples	• 1 finger width below nipple line
• Method	• Heel of 1 hand, other hand on top	• Heel of 1 hand	• 2 fingers
• Depth	• $1^1/_2$ inch to 2 inches	• 1 to $1^1/_2$ inches	• $^1/_2$ to 1 inch
• Rate	• 100 per minute	• 100 per minute	• 100+ per minute
• Ratio of chest compressions to breaths	• 15:2	• 5:1	• 5:1
5. When to activate EMS when alone	Immediately after establishing unresponsiveness	After 1 minute of resuscitation, unless bystander available who can call	After 1 minute of resuscitation, unless bystander available who can call
6. Automated external defibrillation (AED)	Yes	Yes, but requires special electrode pads and reduced energy level.	Yes, but requires special electrode pads and reduced energy level.

Appendix B Automated External Defibrillators (AEDs)

Caring for cardiac arrest

Most sudden cardiac arrest victims have an electrical malfunction of the heart termed ventricular fibrillation. In ventricular fibrillation, the heart's electrical signals, which normally induce a coordinated heartbeat, suddenly become chaotic, and the heart's pumping function abruptly ceases. The victim immediately loses responsiveness, and is considered dead.

Cardiopulmonary resuscitation (CPR) alone will not correct ventricular fibrillation. At best, CPR provides only about 30% of normal blood flow to the brain, and is simply a method to extend the time a victim may remain resuscible.

The best care includes early access, CPR, defibrillation, and advanced care. Defibrillation is often done through the use of automated external defibrillators (AED).

Development of AEDs

Until recently, prehospital defibrillation was a skill reserved for personnel such as paramedics. Advances in computer technology resulted in a new generation of "smart" defibrillators. These devices, called automated external defibrillators (AEDs), are lightweight,

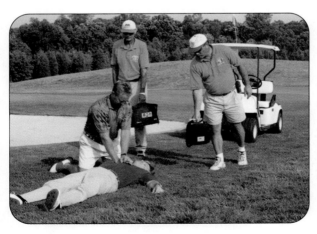

Golf staff arrive to help an apparent heart attack victim.

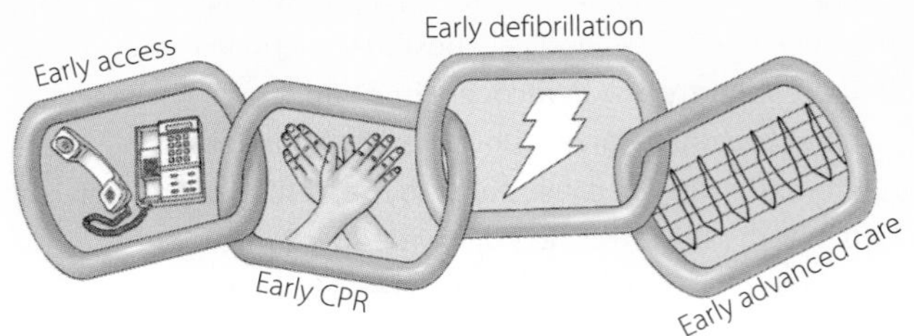

The four links in the chain of survival

can interpret the ECG (heart) rhythm, determine whether defibrillation is required and deliver an electrical shock, when appropriate. The AED guides the operator through every action.

Availability of AEDs

The widespread deployment of AEDs increases survival rates. The strongest determinant of survival in people having an out-of-hospital cardiac arrest is the speed with which shocks are delivered.

Chances of successful resuscitation decreases by about 10% with each minute following sudden cardiac arrest. After 10 minutes, very few resuscitation attempts are successful.

AEDs are readily available on airlines, in airports, at sporting events, in Senior Citizen Centers, and at amusement parks. Other logical locations for an AED include golf courses, and households with high-risk individuals. AED use is being extended beyond healthcare professional and trained emergency personnel to trained citizens. Most states have Public Access Defibrillation (PAD) laws that enable individuals to use AEDs and protect those who help in an emergency situation.

AEDs are easier than CPR

Because of the ease of operation, people can be trained in AED use in a few hours and some say the techniques are easier to learn than CPR. AEDs offer voice prompts which provide operators with clear and concise instructions. New AEDs typically have two buttons: On/Off, and Shock.

Using an AED

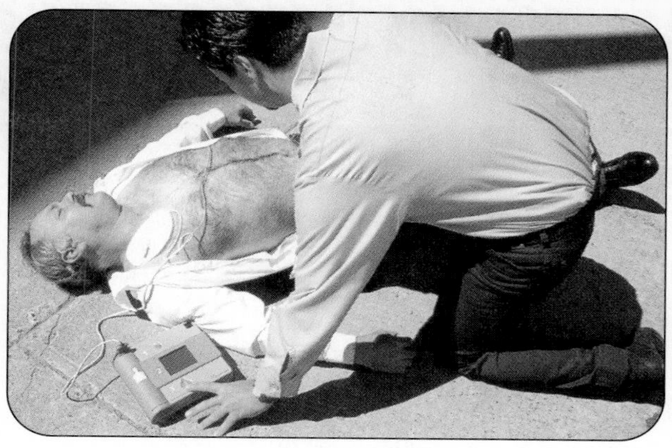

Before AED use, a victim must be– (1) unresponsive, (2) not breathing, (3) without signs of circulation. Once these have been established, the AEDs two pads are attached to the victim to analyze the victim's heart and decide if it is in a shockable rhythm.

If two rescuers are present, one rescuer assesses the victim and begins CPR if necessary. The other rescuer prepares the AED and attaches it to the victim if indicated.

First, turn the unit on. Next, expose the victim's chest and attach the pads. For proper adherence and conduction the skin must be clean and dry. Remove the backing and apply them to the victim's chest. For adults, one pad is placed to the right of the sternum (breastbone) just below the collarbone. The other is placed to the left of the victim's left nipple with the electrode on the side of the chest, above the lower rib margin.

Analyze the heart's rhythm. Make sure no one is touching the victim and the victim is not being moved. These actions could interfere with the analysis. If a shock is indicated, again make sure no one is touching the victim or touching any conductive material in contact with the victim. Once it is safe to do so, press the shock button to deliver the electrical charge.

After delivering the first shock, analyze the rhythm again and repeat the previous steps. Do not check for a pulse until three shocks have been administered or a "No shock indicated" message is displayed. If there is no pulse, perform one minute of CPR. After one minute of CPR, recheck the pulse. If there is still no pulse, analyze the rhythm and deliver up to another three shocks, if indicated. Shocks are administered in sets of three unless a "No shock indicated" message is displayed. AEDs will provide voice and message prompts to guide you through this process.

AEDs and Infants and Children

If signs of circulation are absent in an infant or child, begin CPR until a defibrillator is available. Only about 15% of children in cardiac arrest need defibrillation. Infants and children up to 8 years of age and 55 pounds (25 kg) can be defibrillated with an AED. This requires special equipment and a reduced energy level. There is currently only one AED unit on the market that can be used with infants and children.

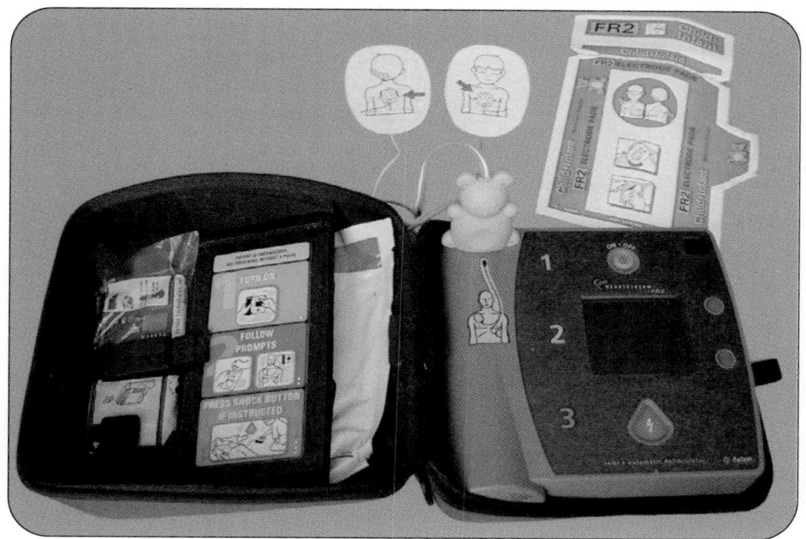

Quick Emergency Index